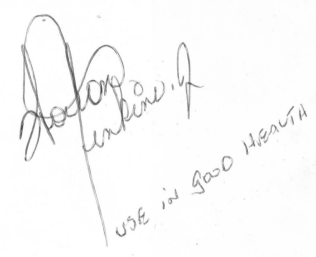

USE IN GOOD HEALTH

# THE DICTIONARY OF VITAMINS

An invaluable reference book giving full, up-to-date information on the complete range of vitamins and vitamin therapy.

# THE DICTIONARY OF VITAMINS

## The Complete Guide to Vitamins and Vitamin Therapy

Compiled and written by
**LEONARD MERVYN**
B.Sc., Ph.D., C.Chem., F.R.S.C.
Member of the New York Academy of Sciences

THORSONS PUBLISHERS INC.
New York

Thorsons Publishers Inc.
377 Park Avenue South
New York, New York 10016

First U.S. Edition 1984

Library of Congress Cataloging in Publication Data

Mervyn, Len.
  The dictionary of vitamins.

  Bibliography: p.
  1. Vitamins—Dictionaries. 2. Vitamin therapy—
Dictionaries. I. Title. [DNLM: 1. Vitamins—
Dictionaries.
2. Vitamins—Therapeutic use—Dictionaries. QU 13
M576d]
QP771.M46    1984      612'.399'0321      84-2465
ISBN 0-7225-0869-7 (pbk.)

Printed and bound in Great Britain

Thorsons Publishers Inc. are distributed to the trade by
Inner Traditions International Ltd., New York

# Dedication

For my daughter Lindsey, and sons
Timothy and Adrian

# Introduction

The first fifty years of the twentieth century saw the concept of accessory food factors put forward by the brilliant researchers Sir Frederick Gowland Hopkins and Casimir Funk and the subsequent isolation of their essential micro-nutrients (called vitamins) by many doctors and scientists who were attracted by the association between these factors and certain diseases. In cases where specific diseases were produced by specific deficiencies of these vitamins, dramatic cures were produced simply by giving these substances or by improving the diet to ensure adequate intakes of them.

In 1954 the concept of inborn errors of metabolism, sometimes hereditary, was introduced when it was observed that certain types of infantile convulsions were responsive to high doses of vitamin $B_6$. These genetically determined disorders increased the individual's vitamin requirements by a factor of 10 to 1000. Why should this happen?

Explanations included:

1. There may be impaired absorption or transport of a vitamin, so increased intake may augment the intake and correct the disorder.
2. Most vitamins require conversion to an active form and the mechanism may be faulty, so the only treatment is to supply the preformed activated vitamin.
3. Those vitamins that function when attached to a specific enzyme may not do so because of an inherent abnormality that precludes them. The answer is often to saturate the enzyme by supplying excessive amounts of the vitamin and cofactor.
4. These enzymes may not survive as long as they should and, by saturating them with the vitamins, their stability is increased.

There are at least 25 vitamin-responsive disorders known that come under the heading of inborn errors of metabolism involving eight water-soluble vitamins and one fat-soluble vitamin. Such diseases are fortunately rare, but clinical response to high-dose vitamins is dramatic.

During the same period, i.e., from the mid-1950s to the present day, there has been a great upsurge in the development of megavitamin therapy, where vitamins are used in doses far higher than needed for their biochemical action, so that they should be regarded more as therapeutic agents. Hence we saw the introduction of B complex for mental disease; vitamin E for heart and blood circulation problems; vitamin C for its anti-infective properties and, in really massive doses, as an adjunct in treating certain cancers.

High doses of vitamins also introduced the increased possibility of side-effects, but with certain exceptions, notably vitamins A and D, these have proved to be largely non-existent and in all cases easily cured by reducing the vitamin intake. Compare these with the side-effects that are guaranteed to occur with any of the medicinal drugs in present-day use.

This dictionary therefore has been written to supply information on the vitamins in a concise though comprehensive manner, to suggest regimes of self-treatment with vitamins that will usually complement the medicinal drugs prescribed by a practitioner, and to answer questions that the author has received from his peers and the public alike during his twenty years involvement with vitamin research and its applications. In the doses recommended the treatments are safe, but if medical supervision is felt to be needed, this is mentioned. Nevertheless it is advisable, when beginning any new health care program, to discuss it with your regular physician or health care practitioner.

Some names of leading researchers both past and present in the field of vitamins have been given. These people must be regarded as the pioneers who had the patience and foresight to discover and isolate these essential micro-nutrients, but they also include those who had the courage to seek new clinical applications for them, often in the face of resistance. It is impossible to include all who have contributed to our knowledge of vitamins; indeed there could be a separate dictionary for these people, but omission in no way diminishes the contribution of all these researchers.

Finally, a note on how quantities of vitamins are expressed, in foods and in supplements. The concept of International Units (IU) is fully explained in the text. In addition, however, it is worth remembering the following relationships:

1 gram       =     1000 milligrams (mg)
1 milligram  =     1000 micrograms ($\mu$g)
100 grams is approximately 3.5 ounces.

# A

**A,** fat-soluble vitamin. Known also as retinol, axerophthol, biosterol. Present in supplements as retinyl palmitate. First isolated in 1913 by two groups of American workers. One microgram is equivalent to 3.33 international units. Found naturally only in foods of animal origin. Anti-infective vitamin.

*Richest sources* are (in μg per 100g): cod liver oil (1800); halibut liver oil (60000); liver (lamb 18100; ox 16500); butter (750); cheeses (up to 385); whole eggs (140). Added to margarine to provide 900μg/100g. Can be manufactured by chemical synthesis.

*Destroyed by* light, high temperatures and air, particularly in the presence of iron and copper (as in utensils).

*Functions* in sight, in maintaining healthy skin and mucous membranes, in resistance to infection, in protein synthesis, in maintaining healthy bones, in preventing anemia and in growth of the young.

*Deficiency in man* leads to: night blindness (inability to see in the dark); xerophthalmia (drying and degenerative disease of the cornea); kidney stone formation; mild skin complaints; inflammation of mucous membranes.

*Deficiency symptoms* include: increased susceptibility to infections of the skin, mucous membranes and respiratory tract; dry, scaly skin and scalp with poor hair quality; poor sight especially under low illumination; burning and itching eyes, inflamed eyelids, headaches and pain in the eyeballs leading to drying and degenerative condition of the eye known as xerophthalmia. Characterized by ulceration and eventually blindness.

*Deficiency in animals* causes dry, scaly skin, poor hair, night blindness, multiple infections, poor absorption, kidney stones, bone overgrowth, sterility, fetal abnormalities.

*Recommended daily intakes* in the USA are 1000μg for men and 800μg for women with additional 200μg during pregnancy and 400μg during lactation. In the UK they vary from 450μg (up to 9 years) to 575μg (9-12 years) to 750µg (12 years to adults) and increase during lactation to 1200µg.

*Highest supplementary intake* permitted in the USA is 25000IU and in the UK is 7500IU per day in medicines available without prescription.

*Toxicity* symptoms include: loss of appetite; dry, itching skin; loss of hair; headaches; nausea and vomiting. Associated with daily intakes as low as 1512µg (5000IU), but ten times this is usually tolerated.

*Alternative* sources of vitamin A are carotenes (*see* separate entry).

*Therapy* with vitamin A essential in night blindness. May be used in cancer, gastric ulcers, acne, eczema and psoriasis.

---

**acetaldehyde,**  toxic substance found in tobacco smoke and produced by body from alcohol. Destroys vitamin $B_1$, vitamin C, vitamin $B_6$. These vitamins plus amino acid L-cysteine can overcome effects of acetaldehyde at dose levels of $B_1$ (10mg), $B_6$ (10mg), vitamin C (500mg), L-cysteine (100mg) daily.

---

**acetylcholine,**  derivative of choline involved in transmission of nerve impulses. Formation depends on adequate vitamin $B_1$, pantothenic acid and choline. Lack of acetylcholine leads to brain damage and may be a factor in senile dementia and Alzheimer's disease.

---

**achlorhydria,**  also known as hypochlorhydria. Lack of production of hydrochloric acid in the stomach. Believed to increase chances of developing gastric cancer. Symptom of pernicious anemia specific to vitamin $B_{12}$ deficiency.

Treat with betaine hydrochloride, also known as lycine hydrochloride; glutamic acid hydrochloride; dilute hydrochloric acid (2ml diluted to 200ml with water and sipped through a straw during meal).

---

**acne,**  inflammation of the hair and sweat glands. Has been treated with oral vitamin A (2272µg or 7500IU daily) plus the mineral zinc (15mg daily as amino acid chelate). Spots may also be treated with cream containing vitamin A or retinoic acid. Also may respond to vitamin F (oil of evening primrose, 500mg capsules, three daily).

Premenstrual flare-up of acne responds to 50mg vitamin $B_6$ daily for one week before menstruation and during it.

---

**Addisonian anemia,**   *See* anemia, pernicious, and $B_{12}$ vitamin.

---

**adrenal,**   gland that produces anti-stress hormones (e.g. cortisol) from cholesterol. High concentration of pantothenic acid and vitamin C in gland needed for production.

---

**ageing,**   increases need for all vitamins, particularly vitamin B complex, vitamin C and vitamin E.

---

**alcohol,**   drinking increases need for whole vitamin B complex but particularly vitamins $B_1$, $B_6$, $B_{12}$ and folic acid plus vitamin C. Acute effects of alcohol drinking prevented by megadoses of vitamin C (1 to 3 grams) plus $B_1$ (10mg), $B_6$ (10mg), $B_{12}$ (10$\mu$g) and folic acid (200$\mu$g). Chronic effects prevented by all vitamins plus vitamin F (oil of evening primrose, 150mg) daily.

---

**almonds,**   kernels provide good quantities of vitamin E and the B vitamins. Vitamin E content is 23mg per 100g. B vitamins present are (in mg per 100g): thiamine 0.24; riboflavin 0.92; nicotinic acid 4.7; pyridoxine 0.10; pantothenic acid 0.47. Folic acid level is 96$\mu$g per 100g; biotin level is 0.4$\mu$g per 100g. Traces only of vitamin C present in almond kernels. When roasted, the thiamine content of almonds is reduced to 0.05mg per 100g; that of pantothenic acid is reduced to 0.25mg per 100g.

---

**alopecia,**   baldness, loss of hair. Symptoms of pantothenic acid deficiency in animals; of biotin deficiency in mink and fox; of vitamin F deficiency.
   May respond to: calcium pantothenate (100mg); biotin (500$\mu$g); wheat germ oil or safflower oil (3-5g); nicotinic acid (35mg); folic acid (200$\mu$g); vitamin $B_{12}$ (5$\mu$g); vitamin E (10IU).

---

**alpha tocopherol,**   *see* E vitamin.

---

**alpha tocopheryl acetate,**   *see* E vitamin.

---

11

**alpha tocopheryl succinate,**   *see* E vitamin.

---

**Alzheimer's disease,**   occurs at any age and is characterized by loss of memory for recent events and an inability to store new memories. *See also* senile dementia. No medical treatment, but some cases respond to 25g lecithin daily, increasing by 25g weekly until side-effects appear (nausea, abdominal bloating, diarrhea), then stopping at previous dose.

Second line of treatment consists of 20g choline chloride daily in 4 doses for 8 weeks, 6 weeks' rest, then 100g lecithin daily in 4 doses for 8 weeks. Memory, language functions and daily living improved. High potency phosphatidyl choline (6 capsules daily) in early stages.

---

**amanitine,**   *see* choline.

---

**amygdalin,**   *see* laetrile.

---

**aminopterin,**   immuno-suppressive agent. Impairs folic acid utilization.

---

**anemia,**   lack of production of normal red blood cells.

*Hemolytic*, due to vitamin E deficiency. In babies, treatment is 10-30IU daily in water-soluble form. In adults arises through malabsorption of fats. Need high doses orally (up to 600IU daily) or moderate doses (up to 200IU) of water-soluble form.

*Iron-deficient*, needs vitamin C (100IU) with each dose of iron supplement.

*Megaloblastic*, needs folic acid but medical diagnosis and treatment essential.

*Pernicious*, responds only to vitamin $B_{12}$. Due to malabsorption of vitamin therefore injection of $B_{12}$ absolutely essential.

*Pyridoxine-deficient*, usually associated with taking contraceptive pill. Prevented by taking 25mg vitamin $B_6$ daily.

*Riboflavin-deficient*, probably caused by reduced activation of folic acid that depends on riboflavin. Prevented by 10mg vitamin $B_2$ daily.

*Sickle cell*, may respond in some cases to vitamin E (450IU) daily.

*Thalassemia* or Mediterranean anemia, may respond to 400-600IU vitamin E daily.

---

**aneurin(e),** *see* vitamin $B_1$

---

**angina,** full name angina pectoris, characterized by severe pain in the chest usually radiating to shoulder and arm. Treated with high doses of vitamin E (800IU and up, depending on response). Favorable response to lecithin (15g per day) also reported. Preliminary results using vitamin F from fish oils promising (eicosopentenoic acid and docosahexenoic acid, EPA and DHA 1500mg total daily). All vitamin therapy compatible with existing drug treatments.

---

**animal galactose factor,** *see* orotic acid.

---

**antacids,** gastric acid neutralizers. Prevent absorption of vitamins A and B complex.

---

**antagonists,** substances that neutralize the action of vitamins or immobilize them. May be naturally occurring or produced synthetically. Used in research to induce vitamin deficiency quickly.

Examples are: *Vitamin A* — mineral oil (liquid paraffin). *Vitamin $B_1$* — alcohol; enzyme thiaminase, present in raw fish; antibiotics; excess sugar. *Vitamin $B_2$* — alcohol; antibiotics; oral contraceptives. *Nicotinamide* — alcohol; antibiotics; leucine, amino acid in high concentrations in millet; niacytin, a bound, unabsorbable form in corn and potatoes, liberated only by alkali; excess sugar. *Vitamin $B_6$* — desoxypyridoxine; isoniazid; hydrallazine; penicillamine; levodopa. *Folic acid* — aminopterin; alcohol; oral contraceptives; phenytoin; primidone. *Vitamin $B_{12}$* — oral contraceptives; intestinal parasites; excess folic acid; vitamin $B_{12}$ acids. *Biotin* — antibiotics; sulphonamides; avidin in raw egg-white. *Choline* — alcohol; excess sugar. *Inositol* — antibiotics. *Pantothenic acid* — methyl bromide, used as fumigant in foods; omega-methyl pantothenic acid. *Vitamin D* — mineral oil. *Vitamin E* — oral contraceptives; mineral oil; ferric iron; rancid fats and oils; excessive PUFA. *Vitamin C* — aspirin; corticosteroids; indomethacin; tobacco smoking; alcohol. *Vitamin K* — warfarin, dicoumarol.

---

**antibiotics,** drugs used to combat infectious diseases. Taken orally can destroy "friendly" intestinal bacteria that are providers of some B vitamins and vitamin K. Ill-effects on digestive system relieved by high doses of vitamin B complex. Vitamin K deficiency treated with acetomenaphthone.

**anti-grey-hair factor,** *see* para-aminobenzoic acid.

**antihemorrhagic vitamin,** *see* K vitamin.

**antineuritic vitamin,** *see* $B_1$ vitamin.

**antipellagra vitamin,** *see* nicotinic acid.

**antipernicious anemia vitamin,** *see* $B_{12}$ vitamin.

**antirachitic vitamin,** *see* D vitamin.

**antisterility vitamin,** *see* E vitamin.

**apples,** *eating* variety supplies carotene, vitamin E and B vitamins (apart from $B_{12}$). Vitamin C levels less than those of cooking apples. Carotene content is 30μg per 100g; vitamin E 0.2mg per 100g. Levels of B vitamins (in mg per 100g) are: thiamine 0.04; riboflavin 0.02; nicotinic acid 0.1; pyridoxine 0.03; pantothenic acid 0.10. Folic acid present at 5μg per 100g; biotin at 0.3μg per 100g. Content of vitamin C is 3mg per 100g.

*Cooking* variety. Minimal losses of all vitamins present in raw state when baked or stewed. Carotene present for all three states (in μg per 100g) is respectively 30, 30 and 25. Vitamin E content at 0.2mg per 100g. B vitamins present are (in mg per 100g), for raw, baked and stewed respectively: thiamine 0.04, 0.03, 0.03; riboflavin 0.02, 0.02, 0.02; nicotinic acid 0.1, 0.1, 0.1; pyridoxine 0.03, 0.02, 0.02; pantothenic acid 0.10, 0.09, 0.08. Folic acid levels are only 5, 3 and 2μg per 100g. Biotin constant at 0.2μg per 100g. Vitamin C levels are respectively 15, 14 and 12mg per 100g. Concentrations are slightly reduced if sugar is used in baking and stewing due to slight diluting effect of sugar.

*Varieties* differ in vitamin C levels, as shown in Table 1. There is more vitamin C in the peel of the apples than in the flesh, so whole apples should be eaten.

**Table 1: Differing vitamin C levels in apple varieties**

|  | *mg vitamin C per 100g* | |
| --- | --- | --- |
|  | *Peeled* | *Unpeeled* |
| Cox Orange Pippin | 2 | 5 |
| Granny Smith | 2 | 8 |
| Golden Delicious | 3 | 10 |
| Sturmer Pippin | 20 | 30 |

**apricots,** *fresh, raw* state (without pits) contribute good amounts of carotene at 1.5mg per 100g (range 1.0-2.4mg) but no vitamin E. B vitamins present (in mg per 100g) are: thiamine 0.04; riboflavin 0.05; nicotinic acid 0.6; pyridoxine 0.07; pantothenic acid 0.30. Folic acid level is 5µg per 100g; but no biotin detected. Vitamin C content is 7mg per 100g.

*Stewed* apricots (without pits) contribute good amounts of carotene at 1.18mg per 100g (without sugar) and 1.15mg per 100g (with sugar). B vitamins present (in mg per 100g) are, without and with sugar respectively: thiamine 0.03, 0.03; riboflavin 0.04, 0.04; pantothenic acid 0.23, 0.21. Folic acid level is constant at 2µg per 100g; biotin is absent. Vitamin C content is 5mg per 100g in stewed fruit. If fruit is stewed with the pits, figures are essentially the same.

*See also* dried apricots.

**arrowroot,** the starch granules of the rhizomes of *Maranta arundinacea*. Trace of vitamin E present but completely devoid of carotene and vitamin C. Traces only of thiamine, riboflavin, nicotinic acid, pyridoxine, pantothenic acid, folic acid and biotin. Vitamin C is absent.

**arteriosclerosis,** hardening of the arteries. Treated with lecithin (15-20 grams daily), vitamin E (400IU twice daily), vitamin C (up to 3 grams daily) and vitamin A (7500IU daily). As preventative treatment, particularly in diabetes, supplement diet with lecithin (5 grams), vitamin E (400IU), vitamin C (500mg) and vitamin A (7500IU) daily.

---

**arthritis,** *rheumatoid*, inflammation of the joints. *Osteo*, degenerative joint disease characterized by calcified out-growths from cartilage.

Rheumatoid arthritis may respond to calcium pantothenate with regime of 500mg daily for 2 days; 1000mg for 3 days; 1500mg for 4 days and 2000mg per day thereafter for a period of 2 months or until relief is obtained. Daily intake is then the minimum needed to maintain relief.

Rheumatoid and osteo arthritis may respond to vitamin C, 4000mg daily in divided doses. Both types of arthritis may respond to high doses (3-6g daily) of nicotinamide (preferred) or nicotinic acid. Supplementary preventative intakes are 100mg calcium pantothenate, 500mg vitamin C and 100mg nicotinamide daily.

---

**ascorbic acid,** *see* C vitamin.

---

**artichokes,** when boiled, supply vitamin A in the form of carotene, 40-90µg per 100g. Traces (0.2mg) only of vitamin E. Small quantities of the vitamin B complex present, apart from vitamin $B_{12}$, at concentrations (in mg per 100g) of: thiamine 0.03-0.10; riboflavin 0.01-0.03; nicotinic acid 0.3-1.1; pyridoxine 0.02-0.07; pantothenic acid 0.07-0.21. Traces of biotin and folic acid present. Some vitamin C present at 2-8mg per 100g.

---

**asparagus,** when boiled, is good source of carotene at 500µg per 100g. Also supplies vitamin E at 2.5mg per 100g. B vitamins present (in mg per 100g) include: thiamine 0.10; riboflavin 0.08; nicotinic acid 1.4; pyridoxine 0.04; pantothenic acid 0.13. Folic acid (30µg) and biotin (0.4µg per 100g) also present. Good source of vitamin C at a level of 200mg per 100g.

---

**aspirin,** analgesic and temperature-reducing drug. Reduces vitamin C body levels by destruction and excessive excretion. Causes gastric bleeding. All side-effects of aspirin can be reduced by taking 100mg vitamin C with each tablet. Also improves absorption of aspirin. Impairs thiamine and folic acid utilization.

---

**asthma,** respiratory disease characterized by attacks of difficult breathing with a feeling of constriction and suffocation. Treatment with vitamin $B_6$ effective in some children and adults. Usual dose is 100mg twice daily. Once relief is obtained (usually after one month) maintenance dose can be lower depending on individual. More likely to help $B_6$-dependent children. Can be taken with all anti-asthmatic drugs. Vitamin C can also help some asthmatics by reducing symptoms of attack. Usual dose 1 gram orally every six hours.

---

**atherosclerosis,** fat deposition within the walls of the arteries causing constriction of the blood vessel.

Treatment with vitamin F as vegetable oils, margarine (PUFA) and soy lecithin. Avoid saturated animal fats. Also vitamin $B_6$ (25mg) daily to ensure body synthesis of lecithin plus vitamin C (1000mg) and vitamin E (800IU) daily.

Prevention by replacing animal fats with vegetable oils and margarines and daily intakes of soy lecithin (5g); vitamin $B_6$ (10mg); vitamin C (500mg); and vitamin E (400IU). Recent studies implicate fish oils containing vitamin F in the form of fatty acids EPA and DHA in preventing and treating atherosclerosis (900-1800mg daily).

---

**athletes,** combination of mental and physical stress associated with competition and training increases requirement of vitamins and minerals, as does high calorie intake. Particular requirements for extra vitamin B complex to ensure full use of extra calories; to ensure adequate supply of anti-stress hormones from adrenals; to supply extra pyridoxine required by most female athletes. Vitamin C also essential for production of anti-stress hormones and in ensuring full potential of muscle energy. Vitamin E essential to ensure adequate supply of oxygen to muscles. Similar function also attributed to pangamic acid.

Minimum needs probably met by up to 1500mg vitamin C, 1000IU vitamin E, 150mg pangamic acid and high potency vitamin B complex.

---

**athlete's foot,** dermatophytosis, Tinea Pedis. Characterized by small eruptions between toes with cracking and scaling and caused by various micro-organisms. Can be relieved by dusting affected area with dry vitamin C crystals or powder.

---

**autism,** personality disease in children who become withdrawn and cease to communicate with outside world.

Has been treated with megavitamin therapy including vitamin C (1, 2 or 3g); nicotinamide (1, 2 or 3g); B$_6$ (150-450mg); calcium pantothenate (200mg); plus high-potency B complex preparation daily depending on age of child. Sometimes vitamin B$_6$ alone is sufficient.

---

**avidin,** unique protein in raw egg-white that binds biotin rendering it unavailable for absorption. Cooking eggs destroys avidin and liberates biotin.

---

**avocadoes,** good source of most vitamins. Claimed to contain vitamin D but has not been confirmed. Carotene present is 100μg per 100g; vitamin E is 3.2mg per 100g. B vitamins are (in mg per 100g): thiamine 0.10; riboflavin 0.10; nicotinic acid 1.8; pyridoxine 0.42; pantothenic acid 1.07. Folic acid level is 66μg per 100g, with that of biotin at 3.2μg per 100g. Good source of vitamin C at 15mg per 100g (range 5-30mg).

---

**axerophthol,** *see* A vitamin.

---

# B

---

**B$_1$,** water-soluble vitamin. Member of the vitamin B complex. Known also as thiamin(e) and aneurin(e). Present in supplements as hydrochloride or nitrate. First isolated from rice polishings in 1926 by Drs. B. C. P. Jansen and W. F. Donath.

*Richest food sources* (in mg per 100g) are: dried brewer's yeast (15.6); yeast extract (3.1); unpolished brown rice (2.93); wheat germ (2.00); raw nuts (0.90); pork (0.90); wheat bran (0.89); soy flour (0.75); oatflakes (0.55); wheat grains (0.46); liver (0.32); whole-wheat bread (0.26). Can be manufactured by chemical synthesis.

*Destroyed* rapidly by alkali, e.g. baking powder, soda and by sulphur dioxide (preservative). Most unstable member of the vitamin B complex.

*Main losses* caused by leaching into cooking water and draining from thawed frozen foods, hence can be recovered by utilizing water.

*Functions* as coenzyme in converting carbohydrate into energy in the muscles and in the nervous system.

*Gross deficiency* leads eventually to beriberi, a killing disease very rare in Europe and the West.

*Mild deficiency* causes easy fatigue, loss of appetite, nausea, muscle weakness and digestive upsets. There is irritability, depression, impairment of memory, lack of concentration, then constipation, with abdominal and chest pains followed by tenderness in the calves and tingling and burning in the toes and soles of the feet.

*Deficiency in animals* causes loss of appetite leading to general weakness and death. Fatty degeneration of heart, fast heartbeat, heart failure. Ulcers of digestive tract. Paralysis of central nervous system and degeneration of nerve endings. Lack of sexual development. Skin discoloration.

*Recommended daily intakes* in the USA are: .5-.8mg for children under 9 years; .9-1mg girls 9-18; 1.5mg women 18-75, with additional .2mg during pregnancy and .4mg during lactation; 1-1.4mg boys 9-18; .9-1.5mg men 18-75. In the UK, recommended intakes are related to calorie intakes ($0.096$mg $B_1$ per 240 calories). In boys vary from 0.3mg (under 1 year) to 1.2mg (at 17 years); girls from 0.3mg (under 1 year) to 0.9mg (at 17 years); adults 1.0 (sedentary) to 1.3mg (active); during pregnancy 1.0mg and during lactation 1.1mg extra required.

*Increased intakes* needed on high carbohydrate diets and during pregnancy, lactations, fever, surgery, physical activity and other stress situations. More is needed by alcohol drinkers and those who habitually take antacid preparations. Old people have increased requirements.

*No toxicity* problems when taken orally at levels up to hundreds of milligrams.

*Therapy* with vitamin $B_1$ essential in beriberi. Has been used to improve mental ability in backward children and some adults; as insect repellant; in treating indigestion and in improving heart function in heart disease. Therapy in painful conditions like lumbago, sciatica, trigeminal neuralgia, facial paralysis and optic neuritis (50-600mg daily).

---

$B_2$, water-soluble vitamin, member of the vitamin B complex. Has strong yellow color. Known as riboflavin(e), lactoflavin(e), vitamin G. Isolated from whey by Dr. R. Khun in 1933 after recognition in yeast by Dr. O. Warburg in 1932.

*Richest sources* (in mg per 100g) are: yeast extract (11.0); dried brewer's yeast (4.3); liver (2.0 to 3.0); wheat germ (0.68); cheese (0.19 to 0.50); whole eggs (0.47); wheat bran (0.36); meat (0.16 to 0.28); soy flour (0.31); yogurt (0.26); milk (0.19); green-leaf vegetables (0.25); legumes (0.15).

*Destroyed* readily by heat but only in alkaline solution. Very unstable to light, being converted to lumiflavin, which itself destroys vitamin C. Lost also into cooking fluids by leaching.

*Functions* as coenzymes called flavin mononucleotide (FMN) and flavin dinucleotide (FAD) essential to convert amino acids (from proteins), fatty acids (from fats) and sugars (from starches) into energy with oxygen. Needed for production and repair of body tissues. Maintains healthy mucous surfaces. Catalyses conversion of tryptophane to nicotinic acid.

*Deficiency* does not cause specific disease but *deficiency symptoms* include cracks and sores in the corners of the mouth with inflammation of the tongue and lips. The eyes become bloodshot and develop a burning sensation with feeling of grit under eyelids. Eyes are very sensitive to light and are easily tired. Scaling of the skin around nose, mouth, forehead, ears and scalp with excessive hair loss. Trembling, dizziness, insomnia and slow learning.

*Deficiency in animals* results in failure to grow. Other signs are dermatitis, loss of hair, conjunctivitis, bloodshot eyes, cataracts, anemia, nerve disease and fatty liver. Impaired reproduction with malformed offspring.

*Recommended daily intakes* in the USA are: .8-1.3mg for children under 9 years; 1.3-1.5mg girls 9-18; 1.7mg women 18-75, with additional .3mg during pregnancy and .6mg during lactation; 1.4-2.0mg boys 9-18; 1.3-1.7mg men 18-75. In the UK, intakes range from 0.4mg (babies) to 1.7mg (17-year-old boys) to 1.6mg (girls) to 1.3mg (women), increasing to 1.6mg during pregnancy and 1.8mg during lactation. Similar to WHO.

*Increased intakes* required by alcohol drinkers, tobacco smokers and those taking the contraceptive pill. Extra 20mg needed.

*Toxicity* of riboflavin is virtually unknown and it is used as food-coloring agent.

*Supplements* containing riboflavin cause strong yellow coloration of urine — completely harmless.

*Therapy* with high doses of riboflavin in mouth ulcers, less dramatic response in gastric and duodenal ulcers. Used to treat ulceration of the cornea of the eye and sometimes cataracts.

---

**B$_6$,** water-soluble vitamin, member of the vitamin B complex. Known as pyridoxine but also exists as pyridoxal and pyridoxamine — all equally active. Present in supplements as pyridoxine hydrochloride and pyridoxine phosphate. Anti-depression vitamin. Isolated from liver by Professor Paul Gyorgy at the University of Pennsylvania, USA, in 1934.

*Richest sources* (in mg per 100g) are: dried brewer's yeast (4.20); wheat bran (1.38); yeast extract (1.30); wheat germ (0.92); oatflakes (0.75); pig liver (0.68); soy flour (0.57); bananas (0.51); wheat grains (0.50); nuts (0.50); meats (0.25 to 0.45); fatty fish (0.45); brown rice (0.42); white fish (0.33); potatoes (0.25); green-leaf vegetables (0.16); legumes (0.16); root vegetables (0.15); whole-wheat bread (0.14); eggs (0.11); dried fruits (0.10). Probably produced by intestinal bacteria. Pyridoxine is commonest in vegetable foods. Pyridoxine and pyridoxamine are usual forms in animal foods.

*Deficiency* causes convulsions in infants and induces depression, anemia and skin complaints in adults. May be related to atherosclerosis, premenstrual syndrome, asthma, kidney stones. No specific disease associated with deficiency.

*Deficiency symptoms* include scaly skin about the eyes, nose and mouth with splitting of the lips and inflammation of the tongue. Peripheral neuritis (inflammation and degeneration of nerve endings) and sometimes migraine. Mild depression, irritability, tiredness, breast discomfort, swollen abdomen, puffy fingers and ankles associated with premenstrual syndrome.

*Dependency* states which may respond to high intakes, impossible to obtain from the diet, include asthma, urticaria, mental retardation, premenstrual tension, convulsions, anemia.

*Deficiency in animals* causes loss of appetite, poor utilization of food, weight loss, vomiting, diarrhea; scaling of the skin around the ears, paws, snout and tail; paralysis of the hind-quarters, uncoordinated muscle action; paralysis, convulsions; brown secretion around the eyes, weakening vision, blindness. In monkeys there is arteriosclerosis similar to that in people; also dental caries develops.

*Recommended daily intakes* in the USA are: for infants (0.3 to 0.6mg); children 1 to 4 (0.9 to 1.8mg); adult males (2.0 to 2.2mg); adult females (2.0mg); during pregnancy 2.6mg; during lactation 2.7mg. Intakes have not been set in the UK or WHO.

*Increased intakes* required by those taking contraceptive pill; women just before their periods; those with morning sickness and diabetes induced by pregnancy; anyone on high-protein diets; those taking the drugs isoniazid, hydralazine, penicillamine (NOT penicillin); oestrogens (as in the contraceptive pill and hormone replacement therapy); alcohol drinkers; tobacco smokers.

*Toxicity* is very low so intakes up to 200mg daily are quite safe. No official limit in supplements. *Incompatible* with anti-Parkinson drug Levodopa.

*Therapy* with pyridoxine effective in premenstrual syndrome; in depression induced by contraceptive pill; in morning sickness; in travel sickness; in radiation sickness; as antidote to hydrazine poisoning; in infantile convulsions; in skin lesions of mouth, nose, lips and face; in anemia; in bronchial asthma; in kidney stones; as diuretic; in skin allergies.

---

**B$_{12}$**,   contains cobalt, hence known as cobalamin. Water-soluble vitamin. Member of vitamin B complex. Known also as anti-pernicious anaemia factor; cyanocobalamin; hydroxocobalamin; LLD factor; aquacobalamin; extrinsic factor; animal protein factor. Present in supplements as: cyanocobalamin; hydroxocobalamin acetate; hydroxocobalamin hydrochloride. Deep red crystalline substance. Last true vitamin to be discovered. Isolated from liver in 1948 by Dr. E. Lester Smith in the UK almost simultaneously with Dr. K. Folkers in the USA. Now obtained commercially by fermentation. Only the natural form available because of complicated structure.

*Richest food sources* (in μg per 100g) are: pig liver (25); pig kidney (14); fatty fish (5); pork (3); beef (2); lamb (2); white fish (2); eggs (2); chicken (0.5); cheeses (0.5 to 1.5); yogurt (0.1); cow's milk (0.3). Presence in foods confined to those of animal origin with exception of spirulina (200). *Stored* in liver which contains up to 2mg per kg.

*Absorption from food* requires presence of intrinsic factor produced by normal stomach. Complex of B$_{12}$ — intrinsic factor absorbed only in the ileum (part of small intestine), with the aid of calcium (usually to a maximum of 5μg). Only 1 per cent of oral intake absorbed by simple diffusion.

*Stable* to cooking methods, but boiling in the presence of alkali can cause losses.

*Functions* in the form of two coenzymes, 5-deoxyadenosyl cobalamin and methylcobalamin. Methylcobalamin acts as carrier of methyl group from methyl tetrahydrofolate (active form of folic acid) to important metabolites in body. Hence needed for synthesis of DNA (deoxyribonucleic acid), the basis of body cell production, particularly that of red blood cells. Functions also in metabolism of fatty acids in maintaining myelin sheath, the insulation layer of nerves. Methyl groups used to produce methionine (amino acid) and choline. Also creatine, necessary for energy reserve in muscles. Hydroxocobalamin functions in detoxification of cyanide introduced in food and tobacco smoke.

*Deficiency in man* causes specifically pernicious anemia, or Addisonian anemia.

*Deficiency symptoms* are those typical of anemia and, more specifically, smooth, sore tongue and nerve degeneration causing tremors, psychosis, mental deterioration; menstrual disorders; excessive pigmentation of the hands that affects only black people.

*Deficiency in animals* causes retarded growth in all species. Pigs and calves develop nervous disorders such as uncoordinated muscle movement, excitability, and tender hind legs. Coat becomes tough and dermatitis develops. Low hatchability of eggs in poultry. All develop anemia.

*Recommended dietary intakes* in the USA are: $3.0\mu g$ for children under 4 years; $6.0\mu g$ for anyone over 4 years; and $8.0\mu g$ for pregnant and lactating women. The WHO recommends: $0.3\mu g$ for babies; 0.9 for children 1 to 3 years; $1.5\mu g$ for children 4 to 9 years; and $2.0\mu g$ for all others, except $3.0\mu g$ for pregnant and lactating women. Recommended intakes have not been set in the UK.

*Supplementation* limited to $10\mu g$ daily in UK for products on general sale.

*Increased requirements* by those suffering from malabsorption (e.g. sprue); by anyone with intestinal parasites; by alcohol drinkers; by heavy smokers; by vegetarians and vegans; by geriatric patients; during pregnancy.

*Toxicity* is virtually unknown. Occasional allergic reaction but only from injections.

*Legislative control* of $B_{12}$ in UK is not for toxicity reasons but because high oral intakes interfere with diagnostic techniques for pernicious anemia.

*Therapy* is specific for pernicious anemia. Must be given by intramuscular injection. Used for moodiness, poor memory, paranoia, mental confusion, neuritis mainly in the aged but sometimes in the young. Used for simple tiredness, muscle fatigue, in providing extra energy, in improving appetite, as general tonic.

---

**$B_{12}b$,**  hydroxocobalamin.

---

**$B_{12}c$,**  nitritocobalamin.

---

**B complex,**  mixture of the B vitamins that tend to occur together in foods of animal, plant and micro-organism origin. Strictly speaking complex consists of eight members: thiamine ($B_1$), riboflavin ($B_2$), nicotinic acid ($B_3$), pantothenic acid ($B_5$), pyridoxine ($B_6$), biotin, folic acid and $B_{12}$, all of which are true vitamins. Some authorities include choline and inositol which can, however, be synthesized by the body.

PABA, pangamic acid, orotic acid and laetrile are part of the B complex in foods but are regarded as factors not vitamins.

---

**backache,**   when due to spinal disc injuries can be relieved or prevented by vitamin C (100mg, three times daily) or possibly more, up to 2000mg daily.

---

**bacon,**   all types of the cooked variety contain only insignificant traces of vitamins A, D and carotene. Vitamin E content ranges from 0.06 to 0.21mg per 100g depending upon method of cooking and type of joint or slices. Very little vitamin $B_{12}$, folic acid and biotin present but good source of the other B vitamins. Concentrations (in mg per 100g) are in range: thiamine 0.34-1.00; riboflavin 0.15-0.24; nicotinic acid 6.4-11.8; pyridoxine 0.24-0.33; pantothenic acid 0.3-0.6.

Completely devoid of vitamin C. Lower end of ranges are associated with the fattier types and on the extent of pre-soaking, which removes water-soluble vitamins.

---

**bacterial vitamin H,**   *see* para-aminobenzoic acid.

---

**baked beans,**   in tomato sauce contain no vitamins A, D and carotene, but 1.4mg vitamin E per 100g is present. B vitamins present (in mg per 100g) are: thiamine 0.07; riboflavin 0.05; nicotinic acid 1.3; pyridoxine 0.12; pantothenic acid absent. Some folic acid present (29µg per 100g) but no biotin. Negligible vitamin C present.

---

**baker's yeast,**   Saccharomyces cerevisae. *Fresh, compressed variety* contains following vitamins (in mg per 100g); carotene (trace); thiamine (0.71); riboflavin (1.7); nicotinic acid (13.0); pyridoxine (0.6); folic acid (1.25); pantothenic acid (3.5); biotin (0.06); vitamin C (trace); vitamin E (trace).

*Dried variety* contains following vitamins (in mg per 100g): carotene (trace); thiamine 2.33; riboflavin 4.0; nicotinic acid 43.0; pyridoxine 2.0; folic acid 4.0; pantothenic acid 11.0; biotin 0.2; vitamin C (trace); vitamin E (trace).

Rich source of RNA and DNA, which together account for 12 per cent of dried yeast.

---

**bananas,**   edible part only. In the raw state carotene level is 200µg per 100g; vitamin E is 0.2mg per 100g. B vitamins present are (in mg per 100g): thiamine 0.04; riboflavin 0.07; nicotinic acid 0.8; pyridoxine 0.51; pantothenic acid 0.26. Folic acid level is 22µg per 100g but biotin is absent. Useful source of vitamin C at 10mg per 100g.

---

**barbiturates,**   sedatives and tranquillizers. Enhance excretion and metabolism of vitamin C levels and reduce conversion of vitamin D to 25-hydroxy vitamin D.

---

**Barcelona nuts,**   supply only thiamine and nicotinic acid in the kernels. B vitamins present are 0.11mg thiamine and 3.1mg nicotinic acid per 100g. Traces of vitamin C present.

---

**barley,**   pearl, in the raw state is completely devoid of carotene. Vitamin E content is 0.5mg per 100g. When boiled, this is reduced to a trace, and the concentrations of all vitamins present are reduced, mainly because of water uptake. B vitamins present are (in mg per 100g), for raw pearl barley and the boiled variety respectively: thiamine 0.12, trace; riboflavin 0.05, trace; nicotinic acid 4.8, 1.7; pyridoxine 0.22, trace; pantothenic acid 0.5, 0.2. Folic acid levels are (in µg per 100g), for the raw and boiled pearl barley, 20 and 3 respectively. Traces only of biotin present in both forms. Vitamin C is absent.

---

**Barton-Wright, E.C.,**   British biochemist who was first to associate rheumatoid arthritis with pantothenic acid deficiency and instigated clinical work proving its effectiveness in 1963.

---

**beans,**   show wide variations in vitamin content depending on type of bean. *See* individual variety.

---

**bean sprouts,** canned variety are devoid of vitamins A, D, E and carotene. Poor source of B vitamins with levels (in mg per 100g) of: thiamine 0.02; riboflavin 0.03; nicotinic acid 0.5; pyridoxine 0.03; pantothenic acid not detected. Traces only of folic acid (12µg per 100g) and biotin. When canned, provide only 1mg vitamin C per 100g; when fresh, vitamin C level is 30mg.

---

**bed sores,** decubitus ulcers or pressure sores. Healing rate increased with vitamin C (500mg daily).

---

**beef,** all cuts when cooked contain traces only of vitamins A, D and carotene. Vitamin E levels (in mg per 100g) range from 0.29 to 0.55. Poor sources of thiamine, folic acid and biotin. Concentrations (in mg per 100g) of other B vitamins are in ranges: thiamine 0.04-0.09; riboflavin 0.24-0.40; nicotinic acid 9.2-12.7; pyridoxine 0.24-0.33; pantothenic acid 0.5-0.9; (in µg per 100g) vitamin $B_{12}$ 1-2; folic acid 8-17.

Higher potencies associated with leaner cuts. Completely devoid of vitamin C. *See also* Meats: Cooking losses.

---

**beef extract,** richest source of the B vitamins but devoid of carotene, vitamin E and vitamin C. B vitamins present are (in mg per 100g): thiamine 9.1; riboflavin 7.4; nicotinic acid 85; pyridoxine 0.53. Folic acid level is 1040µg per 100g; vitamin $B_{12}$ content is 8.3µg per 100g.

---

**beer,** beers and lagers of all kinds, whether bottled or draft, provide useful quantities of the B vitamins (apart from thiamine), including vitamin $B_{12}$ which has been produced by the fermenting micro-organism. Fat-soluble vitamins are absent although there is a trace of carotene in all types. B vitamins present are (in mg per 100ml): thiamine, traces only; riboflavin (range 0.02-0.06); nicotinic acid (range 0.39-1.20); pyridoxine (range 0.012-0.042); pantothenic acid 0.10. Folic acid level is in the range 4-9µg per 100ml; biotin level is constant at 1µg per 100ml. Vitamin $B_{12}$ is present in the range 0.11-0.37µg per 100ml. All beers and lagers are devoid of vitamin C.

---

**beets,** little difference in vitamin contents between raw and boiled. When boiled, devoid of vitamins A, D, E and carotene. Poor source of B vitamins with levels (in mg per 100g) of: thiamine 0.02; riboflavin 0.04; nicotinic acid 0.4; pyridoxine 0.03; pantothenic acid 0.10. Reasonable source of folic acid at level of $50\mu g$ per 100g but only traces of biotin are present. Vitamin C is only 5mg per 100g.

**beriberi,**   disease due specifically to lack of vitamin $B_1$. Characterized by loss of mental alertness, respiratory problems and heart damage. Early symptoms are fatigue, loss of appetite, nausea, muscle weakness, digestive upsets. Mental symptoms include depression, irritability, impairment of memory, loss of powers of concentration. Water retention leading to heart and circulation problems. Therapy with 25mg vitamin $B_1$ daily.

**beta tocopherol,**   *see* E vitamin.

**bilberries,**   in the raw state carotene level is $130\mu g$ per 100g but no vitamin E detected. B vitamins present are (in mg per 100g): thiamine 0.02; riboflavin 0.02; nicotinic acid 0.5; pyridoxine 0.06; pantothenic acid 0.16. Folic acid level is $6\mu g$ per 100g but biotin is absent. Good source of vitamin C at 22mg per 100g (range 10-44mg).

**bile acids,**   constituents of bile needed to emulsify fats in digestive process. Produced from cholesterol by the action of vitamin C, so represents main mechanism for reducing blood cholesterol levels.

**bioflavonoids,**   originally called vitamin P. Known also as flavones; bioflavonoid complex. Always accompany vitamin C in natural foods. Water-soluble factors that include: rutin; hesperidin; quercetin; nobiletin; tangeritin; sinensetin; eriodictyol; heptamethoxy flavone; myricetin; kempferol.
   *Richest food sources* are: citrus fruits (skins and pulps); apricots; cherries; grapes; green peppers; tomatoes; papaya; broccoli; cantaloupe; buckwheat. Entire complex present in lemons. Buckwheat richest in rutin. Central white core of citrus fruits richest source.
   *Stability* is high, even in canned fruits and vegetables.
   *Functions* with vitamin C in maintaining the integrity of blood vessels

particularly the capillaries; as anti-inflammatory agents; as anti-infective agents.

*Deficiency symptoms* include small hemorrhages under the skin; easy bruising.

*Toxicity* symptoms have not been reported.

*Therapy* found to be beneficial in menstrual problems, particularly functional uterine bleeding; in varicose veins; in varicose ulcers; in hemorrhoids; in excessive bruising especially when associated with sports; in treating thrombosis; in nosebleeds; in bleeding gums. Two types of bioflavonoids with specific and distinct actions:

1  Methoxylated type, occur almost exclusively in citrus fruits. Nobiletin possesses anti-inflammatory action. Other methoxylated bioflavonoids prevent stickiness of platelets and hence thin the blood. Nobiletin and tangeretin act as detoxifying agents. Other methoxylated bioflavonoids possess anti-infective properties.

2  Hydroxylated bioflavonoids like quercetin, myricetin and kempferol appear to prevent cataract formation. Act as anti-oxidants to preserve foods. Rutin specific in treating high blood pressure, arteriosclerosis and hemorrhages under the skin.

---

**bios I,**   *see* inositol.

---

**bios II,**   *see* biotin.

---

**biotin,**   water-soluble vitamin, member of the vitamin B complex. Known as vitamin H; bios II, coenzyme R. Isolated from liver by Dr. Paul Gyorgy in 1941. Natural form is D-biotin.

*Richest sources* (in μg per 100g) are: dried brewer's yeast (80); pig kidney (32); pig liver (27); yeast extract (27); eggs (25); oatflakes (20); wheat bran (14); wheat germ (12); whole-wheat bread (6); corn (6); fatty fish (5); white fish (3); meats (3); unpolished brown rice (3); milk, cheese and yogurt (2); vegetables (0.1 to 0.6). Substantial amounts produced by intestinal bacteria.

*Stable* to cooking methods, most losses due to leaching into cooking water. Serious losses during drying of milk for baby foods.

*Functions* as coenzyme for wide variety of body metabolic reactions. Required for production of energy from carbohydrates, fats and protein and for interconversions. Essential for maintenance of healthy skin, hair, sweat glands, nerves, bone marrow and glands producing sex hormones.

*Deficiency in babies* causes seborrhoeic dermatitis and desquamative erythroderma (Leiner's disease). No specific deficiency disease in human adults.

*Deficiency symptoms* in babies are dry scaling of the scalp and face with persistent diarrhea. In adults there is fatigue, depression, sleepiness, nausea and loss of appetite. Muscular pains develop and reflexes are lost. Tongue becomes pale and smooth. Mild skin complaints including scaly dermatitis appear. Hair loss. Blood cholesterol levels increase. Specific anemia appears.

*Deficiency* may be induced by excessive intake of raw egg-whites — these contain protein called avidin which immobilizes biotin. Avidin destroyed by cooking.

*Deficiency in animals* causes dermatitis in pigs; impaired growth, dry and brittle feathers, defective bone formation in poultry; dermatitis and blood disorders in rats, plus widespread hair loss, paralysed limbs, weight loss leading to death.

*Recommended dietary intakes* have not been set in UK, USA or WHO since intakes are considered sufficient and intestinal synthesis cannot be assessed. Daily intake from diet calculated at 150 to 400μg.

*Increased intakes* needed on antibiotic therapy; in the new-born child on dried milks; during stress situations.

*Toxicity* is unknown. Babies have received 10mg daily with no adverse effects.

*Therapy* has been successful in seborrheic dermatitis; Leiner's disease; alopecia; scalp disease; skin complaints. Given to babies to prevent crib death.

---

**birth defects,** some can be associated with vitamin deficiencies in mother. Pantothenic acid deficiency can cause still births, premature births, malformed babies and mentally retarded babies. Riboflavin deficiency can cause congenital malformations including cleft palate.

Folic acid deficiency has been implicated in neural tube defects leading to spina bifida.

---

**biscuits,** *homemade* variety contain vitamins A and E in addition to B vitamins, providing (in mg per 100g): thiamine 0.14; riboflavin 0.06; nicotinic acid 2.0; pyridoxine 0.07; folic acid 0.007; pantothenic acid 0.3; biotin 0.004; vitamin A 0.24; vitamin E 2.2.

*Shortbread* variety contain vitamins A, D and E in addition to B vitamins, providing (in mg per 100g): thiamine 0.15; riboflavin 0.01; nicotinic acid 2.4; pyridoxine 0.07; folic acid 0.007; vitamin A 0.23; carotene 0.14; vitamin E 0.6; vitamin D 0.23$\mu$g.

---

**Bishop, K. S.,**  American scientist. *See* H. M. Evans.

---

**blackberries,**  some small loss of vitamins when raw fruit is stewed, with or without sugar. Carotene content (in $\mu$g per 100g), for raw and stewed fruit respectively, is 100 and 85. Vitamin E levels are 12.7 and 2.7mg per 100g respectively. Cultivated blackberries contain 2.7mg per 100g in the raw state. B vitamins present are (in mg per 100g), for raw and stewed fruit respectively: thiamine 0.03, 0.02; riboflavin 0.04, 0.03; nicotinic acid 0.5, 0.5. Biotin levels are 0.4 and 0.3$\mu$g per 100g respectively; folic acid has not been detected. Vitamin C contents are 20 and 14mg per 100g for raw and stewed blackberries respectively.

---

**black currants,**  one of the richest sources of vitamin C, but also provide other vitamins. All concentrations reduced by stewing, with and without sugar. Carotene levels are (in $\mu$g per 100g), for raw and stewed fruit respectively, 200 and 170. Vitamin E levels are 1.0 and 0.9mg per 100g respectively. B vitamins present are (in mg per 100g), for raw and stewed fruit respectively: thiamine 0.03, 0.02; riboflavin 0.06, 0.05; nicotinic acid 0.4, 0.3; pyridoxine 0.08, 0.06; pantothenic acid 0.4, 0.3. Biotin present at concentration of 2.4 and 2.0$\mu$g per 100g respectively for raw and stewed fruit; folic acid is absent. Vitamin C content reduced from 200mg (range 150-230mg) per 100g to 150mg when black currants are stewed. Canned black currants contain 100mg vitamin C per 100g.

---

**blindness,**  night, characterized by an inability to see in the dark. Specific result of vitamin A deficiency. Prevented and cured by vitamin A (2500-7500IU daily).

---

**blood,**  vitamins required for healthy blood production include B$_{12}$, folic acid, E, C and B$_6$.

---

**blood clot,** thrombosis. In heart, coronary thrombosis. In brain, cerebral thrombosis or stroke. Supplement with vitamin E (400-800IU daily) and lecithin (15g daily). Medical treatment includes vitamin K antagonists, e.g. warfarin.

---

**blood-pressure,** usually measured at two levels; higher is systolic, maximum pressure of heart contraction; lower is diastolic, resting heart pressure. Hypertension regarded as diastolic pressure greater than 90mm.

High blood-pressure may respond to choline (up to 1000mg per day) itself; as lecithin (up to 15g per day). Claims also that rutin (up to 600mg daily) can help reduce high blood-pressure.

---

**bone,** normal development and healthy maintenance need vitamin D and vitamin A at minimum daily intakes of 250IU and 2500IU respectively.

*Bone pain* of cancer has been relieved with very high doses (up to 10g daily) of vitamin C.

---

**brains,** provide traces only of vitamins A, D and carotene, but vitamin E ranges from 1.1 to 2.3mg per 100g. B vitamins concentrations (in mg per 100g) are: thiamine 0.08-0.10; riboflavin 0.19-0.24; nicotinic acid 4.6-4.9; pyridoxine 0.08-0.12; pantothenic acid 1.4; vitamin $B_{12}$ 8.0$\mu$g. Poor source of folic acid (3-6$\mu$g) and biotin (3$\mu$g). Vitamin C levels are 17mg per 100g. Levels vary slightly between boiled calf and lamb's brains.

---

**bran,** from wheat, rich source of B vitamins providing (in mg per 100g): thiamine 0.89; riboflavin 0.36; nicotinic acid 32.6; pyridoxine 1.36; pantothenic acid 2.4; folic acid 0.260; biotin 0.014; vitamin E 2.6. Devoid of vitamins A, D, C and carotene.

---

**Brazil nuts,** kernels are good source of B vitamins and vitamin E. Vitamin E level is 17.5mg per 100g. B vitamins present are (in mg per 100g): thiamine 1.00; riboflavin 0.12; nicotinic acid 4.2; pyridoxine 0.17; pantothenic acid 0.23. Folic acid and biotin are virtually absent. Traces only of vitamin C present in Brazil nuts.

---

**bread,** *whole-wheat*, provides fewer B vitamins than whole-wheat flour because of losses due to baking and presence of extra water, providing (in mg per 100g): thiamine 0.26; riboflavin 0.06; nicotinic acid 5.6; pyridoxine 0.14; folic acid 0.039; pantothenic acid 0.6; biotin 0.006; vitamin E 0.2.

*White* provides fewer B vitamins than whole-wheat bread, providing (in mg per 100g): thiamine 0.18; riboflavin 0.03; nicotinic acid 3.0; pyridoxine 0.04; folic acid 0.027; pantothenic acid 0.3; biotin 0.001; vitamin E, trace.

**breast disease,** *see* cancer and cysts.

**brewer's yeast,** *Saccharomyces cerevisae*. Dried variety contains following vitamins (in mg per 100g): carotene (trace); thiamine (15.6); riboflavin (4.28); nicotinic acid (37.9); pyridoxine (4.2); pantothenic acid (9.5); biotin (0.08); folic acid (2.4); vitamin C (trace).

Rich source of RNA and DNA, which together account for 12 per cent of dried yeast. *See also* yeast extract.

**broad beans,** when boiled supply 250µg carotene per 100g and 2.5mg vitamin E. B vitamins include (in mg per 100g): thiamine 0.10; riboflavin 0.04; nicotinic acid 3.7; pyridoxine, not detected; pantothenic acid 3.8. Supplies traces only of folic acid and biotin. Good source of vitamin C at 15mg per 100g, which is reduced to 6mg in canned variety.

**broccoli tops,** rich source of carotene (2.5mg per 100g) but vitamin E levels only 1.1mg per 100g in boiled variety. All B vitamins are reduced when broccoli tops are boiled. Levels are as follows, raw figures first (in mg per 100g): thiamine 0.10, 0.06; riboflavin 0.3, 0.2; nicotinic acid 1.6, 1.2; pyridoxine 0.21, 0.13; pantothenic acid 1.0, 0.7. Levels of folic acid and biotin are respectively (in µg per 100g): 130, 120; 0.5, 0.3. Drastic reduction in vitamin C concentration in boiling, from 110 to 34mg per 100g.

**bronchitis,** inflammation of the bronchial tubes. Vitamin A (7500IU daily) helps in therapy by stimulating the mucous membrane of the respiratory tract to resist infection. Vitamin C (500-1000mg daily) increases resistance to bacterial and viral infections.

---

**bruises,**  hemorrhages under the skin due to capillary fragility. Color changes related to conversion of blood hemoglobin to bile pigments. Excessive bruising prevented by adequate intakes of vitamin C plus bioflavonoids, particularly in persons involved in body contact sports.

---

**Brussels sprouts,**  good source of carotene at 0.4mg per 100g. Vitamin E level is 0.9mg per 100g. All B vitamins are lost when Brussels sprouts are boiled. Levels are as follows, raw figures first (in mg per 100g): thiamine 0.10, 0.06; riboflavin 0.15, 0.10; nicotinic acid 1.5, 0.9; pyridoxine 0.28, 1.17; pantothenic acid 0.4, 0.28. Levels of folic acid and biotin are respectively (in $\mu$g per 100g): 110, 87; 0.4, 0.3. Vitamin C concentration reduced from 90 to 40mg per 100g when boiled.

---

**bruxism,**  grinding of the teeth, often carried on during sleep, that can give rise to dental problems. Has been overcome by increasing intake of calcium pantothenate (100mg) and calcium (300mg) daily.

---

**burns,**  infection and pain of burn area of skin reduced by spray of 3 per cent vitamin C solution (sterile). Healing rate increased by massive doses (up to 10g) of vitamin C orally. Complemented by simultaneous intake of 400IU vitamin E twice daily plus vitamin E cream or ointment (100IU per gram).

---

**butter,**  salted. Good source of fat-soluble vitamins but negligible quantities of water-soluble vitamins present. Provides (in $\mu$g per 100g): vitamin A 750; carotene 470; vitamin D 0.76; vitamin E 2000.

---

**butter beans,**  also called Lima beans. Virtually devoid of fat-soluble vitamins. B vitamins present include (in mg per 100g): thiamine 0.45; riboflavin 0.13; nicotinic acid 5.6; pyridoxine 0.58; pantothenic acid 1.0. Good source of folic acid at 110$\mu$g per 100g. No vitamin C present.

---

# C

**C,** water-soluble vitamin. Known also as L-ascorbic acid; anti-scorbutic acid; hexuronic acid; cevitannic acid; L-xyloascorbic acid; ascorbyl palmitate; ascorbyl nicotinate. White crystalline powder. Isolated from fruits, paprika and adrenal glands by Dr. Albert Szent-Gyorgi in 1922 in Hungary. Shown in 1932 by Dr. Szent-Gyorgi and Drs. W. A. Waugh and C. G. King (USA) that substance cured scurvy.

*Richest food sources* (in mg per 100g) are: acerola cherry juice (3390); camu pulp (2994); rose-hip syrup (295); black currants (200); guavas — raw (200); guavas — canned (180); parsley (150); kale (150); horseradish (120); broccoli tops (110); green peppers (100); tomato purée (100); Brussels sprouts (90); chives (80); lemons (80) — juice (50); cauliflower (60); watercress (60); strawberries (60); Savoy cabbage (60); red cabbage (55); winter cabbage (55); oranges (50) — juice (50); mustard tops (50); white cabbage, mustard and cress, blackberries, gooseberries, grapefruit, lychees (all 40); all other fruits and vegetables (20 to 35) except lettuce, apples, avocadoes, quinces (15); sweet corn (12); bananas, rhubarb, onion (10); cod roe (30); meats (7 to 23); fish, cow's milk (1.5).

*Unstable* in cooking methods and food processing. Destroyed and lost by leaching into cooking water. High temperature (e.g. pressure cooking), short time, small volume of water best conditions for retention. Soaking vegetables to be avoided. Freeze-drying preserves vitamin C; hot air drying causes wholesale destruction; gross losses caused by oxygen, light, heat, alkalis in presence of copper. Deep, really hot, frying preferred to slow frying in shallow pan.

*Functions* in protective role as anti-oxidant; in promoting iron absorption; in accumulating iron in bone marrow, spleen and liver; in production of collagen, the connective tissue protein of the body; in maintaining resistance to bacterial and viral diseases; in controlling blood cholesterol levels; in converting vitamin folic acid into active form folinic acid; in mutually protecting vitamin E; in production of anti-stress hormones; in converting amino acids to substances needed for normal brain and nerve functions; in tooth and bone formation; in maintaining healthy blood capillaries; in maintaining healthy sex organs; as antihistamine in preventing allergic reactions.

*Deficiency in man* results in scurvy.

*Deficiency symptoms* are lassitude, weakness, irritability, vague muscle and joint pains, loss of weight. Bleeding gums, gingivitis, loosening of the teeth. Minute hemorrhages (bleeding) under the skin. Larger hemorrhages, particularly in thigh muscles. Severe symptoms are hemorrhaging of the eye, brain with bleeding from nose, digestive tract and urinary tract.

*Deficiency in infants* usually shows between six and eighteen months. Infant cries on being handled, is irritable with loss of appetite and thus weight. Tenderness of the extremities, pain on movement. Hemorrhages in long bones, gums, skin, mucous membranes. Thickening at ends of ribs. Cessation of bone formation.

*Deficiency in animals* rare because most can synthesize it from glucose. In guinea pigs and monkeys deficiency produces scurvy and muscle wasting, blood capillary fragility and slow wound healing.

*Recommended dietary intakes* in the USA are: 35mg for babies up to 1 year; 45mg for children 1 to 10 years; 50mg for children 11 to 17 years; and 60mg for anyone over 14, except 80mg for pregnant and 100mg for lactating women. In the UK, intakes are: 20mg for children up to eight years; 25mg for children 9 to 14 years; 30mg for persons 15 to 17 years; and 30mg for all others, except 60mg for pregnant and lactating women. WHO recommendations are similar.

*No limit* on supplementation in the USA or UK.

*Increased requirements* by those under stress; by those taking aspirin, contraceptive pill, tetracycline antibiotics, barbiturates, corticosteroids; by tobacco smokers; by alcohol drinkers; by the elderly; by athletes; by those undergoing operations; by those with infectious diseases; by those injured in accidents; by those undergoing dental surgery; by bottle-fed infants; by those with gastric and duodenal ulcers; by diabetics.

*Extra vitamin C* can be beneficial to increase growth and blood production and to reduce diarrhea in new-born piglets; to increase laying output and eggshell hardness in poultry; to increase sperm production in young cocks; to increase resistance to infection and reduce requirements for group B vitamins in poultry.

*Therapy* specific in treating scurvy. Beneficial results claimed in iron-deficiency anemia; increased capillary fragility giving rise to skin hemorrhage; gastro-intestinal hemorrhages; infectious diseases, particularly those of the respiratory tract; to increase rate of healing after accidental and surgical injury; to treat spongy and bleeding gums; to treat loosened teeth; to treat many psychiatric states; to treat colds and influenza; to prevent and treat cancer; to reduce high blood cholesterol levels; as an antihistamine to reduce allergic reactions; to treat atherosclerosis; to treat arthritis; to treat bed sores; to reduce leg cramps during pregnancy; to treat lead, mercury and cadmium poisoning; to prevent and treat alcoholic hangovers.

**cabbage,** *see* individual variety.

---

**cadmium,** toxic mineral present in high concentration in polluted atmospheres. Vitamin C at daily dose levels of 500-1000mg protects against cadmium poisoning and helps rid body of mineral.

---

**calciferol,** *see* D$_2$ vitamin.

---

**calcium pantothenate,** *see* pantothenic acid.

---

**Cameron, Ewan,** Scottish surgeon, consultant in Vale of Leven Hospital, Scotland, and Research Professor at the Linus Pauling Institute of Science and Medicine in Menlo Park, California, USA. Initiated high potency vitamin C as treatment for cancer.

---

**cancer,** malignant growths that can be treated with high doses of vitamins in addition to conventional therapy.

*Bladder* — needs sufficient vitamin C to saturate urinary system to protect against and treat cancer of the bladder. 500mg three times daily is effective. Inositol (1000mg daily) also has inhibiting effect.

*Breast* — clinical response obtained with 200IU vitamin E three times daily. Simultaneous intake of up to 10g daily vitamin C may complement vitamin E therapy. Dose of C arrived at by increasing intake by 1g each day until diarrhea occurs. One gram per day less than this is maximum tolerated dose up to maximum of 10g.

*Colon* — use vitamin C with same regime as in treating breast cancer.

*Lung* — prevention (particularly in tobacco smokers) and treatment with beta-carotene (4.5mg three times daily).

*Skin* — preliminary reports suggest 0.05 per cent retinoic acid applied directly to skin areas affected has beneficial effect. Other retinoids may be more effective.

*Other cancers* — vitamin C therapy as outlined for breast cancer may be beneficial.

Laetrile claimed to be beneficial in all cancers but professional treatment essential.

---

**canned peas,**   reduced levels of water-soluble vitamins compared to fresh peas, that are reduced even further in processed variety. Carotene and vitamin E concentrations are identical to those of fresh peas, with 0.3mg and 0.9mg per 100g respectively. B vitamins present are (in mg per 100g), for canned and processed peas respectively: thiamine 0.13, 0.10; riboflavin 0.10, 0.04; nicotinic acid 2.8, 1.6; pyridoxine 0.06, 0.03; pantothenic acid 0.15, 0.08. Folic acid level reduced drastically from 52 to 3µg per 100g in canned and processed peas; traces only of biotin. Vitamin C level reduced from 8mg per 100g to only traces.

---

**carnitine,**   constituent of muscles and liver. Synthesis in body dependent on vitamin C. Functions as transporter of fatty acids within body cells prior to using them for energy production.

---

**carotenemia,**   high blood levels of carotene that may cause yellow coloration of the skin. Completely harmless and removed by reducing intake of carotenes. Eyeballs remain white which distinguishes it from jaundice.

---

**carotenoids,**   colored pigments widely distributed in animals and plants. More than 100 identified in nature. Includes carotenes designated alpha-, beta-, and gamma-carotene that can give rise to vitamin A. Cryptoxanthin and beta-zeacarotene are also vitamin A precursors. Conversion takes place in intestine and liver.

*Richest food sources* (in µg per 100g) are: carrots (12000); parsley (7000); spinach (6000); turnip tops (6000); spring greens (4000); sweet potatoes (4000); watercress (3000); broccoli (2500); cantaloupe melons (2000); endives (2000); pumpkin (1500); apricots (1500); lettuce (1000); prunes (1000); tomatoes (600); spring cabbage (500); peaches (500); asparagus (500); ox liver (1540); butter (470); cheese (210); cream (125); cow's milk (22).

*Relationship* between carotenes and vitamin A is as follows:

1 retinol equivalent = 1 microgram retinol
= 6 micrograms beta-carotene
= 12 micrograms other carotene precursors
= 3.33IU vitamin A activity from retinol
= 10IU vitamin A activity from beta-carotene

Beta-carotene is most potent precursor of vitamin A.

*Destroyed* by high temperatures, oxygen and light particularly with traces of iron and copper. Losses of 40 per cent in boiling water (60 mins); 70 per cent in frying (15 mins); freezing and canning and cooking loses 20 per cent; controlled drying of fruits and vegetables causes 20 per cent loss; drying in sun causes virtual complete destruction.

*Functions* of carotenes are as precursors of vitamin A. No other specific function known.

*Deficiency* not known to cause any specific disease.

*Deficiency symptoms* are not known.

*Recommended dietary intakes* have not been set by any authority. Possible to obtain full daily vitamin A requirements from carotenes alone. Usual diets supply 50 per cent vitamin A needs as vitamin and 50 per cent as carotenes.

*Legal limits* of carotene intakes in supplements related to vitamin A, i.e., 2250µg retinol equivalents, in products on general sale.

*Toxicity* has not been reported for carotenes. Symptoms of excess are yellowing of skin that is reversible and harmless.

*Therapy* with beta-carotene claimed to be beneficial in lung cancer in animal tests. Appears to be protective against lung cancer induced by tobacco smoking.

---

**carrots,** *old,* raw carrots contain higher levels of the water-soluble vitamins than the boiled variety. When boiled, both young and old carrots have the same B vitamins content but higher levels of carotene are present in the old. Concentrations present in old carrots, raw figures first (in mg per 100g) are: carotene 12.0, 12.0; vitamin E 0.5, 0.5. B vitamins are: thiamine 0.06, 0.05; riboflavin 0.05, 0.04; nicotinic acid 0.7, 0.5; pyridoxine 0.15, 0.09; pantothenic acid 0.25, 0.18. Folic acid contents are (in µg per 100g) 15, 8; and biotin levels are 0.6, 0.4. Boiling reduces vitamin C content from 6 to 4mg per 100g.

*Young* carrots lose water-soluble vitamins when processed in cans. Fat-soluble are unaffected — carotene is stable for years in canned carrots. Concentrations present in young carrots (boiled and canned respectively, in mg per 100g) are: vitamin A 6.0, 7.0; vitamin E 0.5, 0.5. B vitamins present are: thiamine 0.05, 0.04; riboflavin 0.04, 0.02; nicotinic acid 0.5, 0.4; pyridoxine 0.09, 0.02; pantothenic acid 0.18, 0.10. Folic acid levels are (in µg per 100g) 8.0, 7.0; while biotin levels are 0.4, 0.4. Some reduction of vitamin C content from 4 to 3 mg per 100g after canning process.

---

**cashew nuts,** good source of carotene at 60μg per 100g. Vitamin E present at level of 2.2mg per 100g. B vitamins present are (in mg per 100g): thiamine 0.43; riboflavin 0.25; nicotinic acid 1.8. No other vitamins have been detected.

**cataracts,** opacity of the eye lens. Can be induced by deficiency of vitamins $B_2$ and C and the mineral calcium. May be prevented by vitamin $B_2$ (10mg daily) vitamin C (500mg daily) and clacium (500mg daily).

**cathartics,** purgatives and laxatives. Prevent absorption of vitamin K and riboflavin.

**cauliflower,** some loss of water-soluble vitamins when boiled but little change in carotene and vitamin E levels. Carotene contents are (in mg per 100g) for both raw and boiled cauliflower 0.03; vitamin E reduced from 0.4 to 0.2 on boiling. Levels of B vitamins (in mg per 100g), raw figures first, are: 0.10, 0.06; riboflavin 0.10, 0.06; nicotinic acid 1.1, 0.8, pyridoxine 0.20, 0.12. Reasonable source of folic acid at levels of (in μg per 100g) 39, 49; and of biotin at 1.5, 1.0. Substantial losses of vitamin C from 60 to 20mg per 100g on boiling cauliflower.

**celeriac,** a turnip-rooted variety of celery. Completely devoid of carotene and vitamin E. When boiled, levels of B vitamins are (in mg per 100g): thiamine 0.04; riboflavin 0.04; nicotinic acid 0.8; pyridoxine 0.10. Other B vitamins not detected. Vitamin C concentration is 4mg per 100g.

**celery,** traces only of carotene and level of only 0.2mg per 100g vitamin E in both raw and boiled vegetable. Levels of B vitamins and vitamin C reduced on boiling. Concentrations (in mg per 100g), raw figures first, are: thiamine 0.03, 0.02; riboflavin 0.03, 0.02; nicotinic acid 0.5, 0.3; pyridoxine 0.10, 0.06; pantothenic acid 0.40, 0.28. Traces only of biotin and folic acid. Vitamin C content reduced from 7.0 to 5.0mg per 100g in boiling.

**cephalosporins,** antibiotics. Prevent absorption of vitamins K, $B_{12}$ and folic acid.

---

**chapatis,** useful source of B vitamins when the food is part of the staple diet, providing (in mg per 100g): thiamine 0.26; riboflavin 0.04; nicotinic acid 3.4; pyridoxine 0.21; folic acid 0.015; pantothenic acid 0.3; biotin 0.002. Slightly lower levels when made with fat.

---

**cheese,** supplies most vitamins, mainly derived from milk but some produced by bacterial synthesis during production. All cheeses are devoid of vitamin C.

*Edam and Cheddar types* provide (in mg per 100g): vitamin A 0.31; carotene 0.205; thiamine 0.04; riboflavin 0.50; nicotinic acid 6.22; pyridoxine 0.08; folic acid 0.02; pantothenic acid 0.30; biotin 0.002; vitamin $B_{12}$ 0.0015; vitamin E 0.8; vitamin D 0.26µg.

*Danish Blue type* provides (in mg per 100g): vitamin A 0.27; carotene 0.17; thiamine 0.03; riboflavin 0.60; nicotinic acid 6.32; pyridoxine 0.15; folic acid 0.05; pantothenic acid 2.0; biotin 0.002; vitamin $B_{12}$ 0.0012; vitamin E 0.7; vitamin D 0.23µg.

*Camembert type* provides (in mg per 100g): vitamin A 0.215; carotene 0.135; thiamine 0.05; riboflavin 0.60; nicotinic acid 6.17; pyridoxine 0.20; folic acid 0.06; pantothenic acid 1.4; biotin 0.006; vitamin $B_{12}$ 0.0012; vitamin E 0.6; vitamin D 0.181µg.

*Stilton type* provides (in mg per 100g): vitamin A 0.37; carotene 0.23; thiamine 0.07; riboflavin 0.30; nicotinic acid 6.03; vitamin E 1.0; vitamin D 0.312µg. Others not known.

*Cottage cheese*, poor source of vitamins when compared to the other cheeses, providing (in mg per 100g): vitamin A 0.032; carotene 0.018; thiamine 0.02; riboflavin 0.19; nicotinic acid 3.29; pyridoxine 0.01; folic acid 0.009; vitamin $B_{12}$ 0.5µg; vitamin D 0.0023µg.

*Cream cheese*, good source of fat-soluble vitamins but lower levels of water-soluble vitamins than hard cheeses, providing (in mg per 100g): vitamin A 0.385; carotene 0.22; vitamin E 1.0; thiamine 0.02; riboflavin 0.14; nicotinic acid 0.82; pyridoxine 0.01; folic acid 0.005; vitamin $B_{12}$ 0.3µg; vitamin D 0.275µg.

*Processed cheese* supplies useful quantities of vitamin A and carotene but other vitamins are present in lower concentration than in named cheeses, providing (in mg per 100g): vitamin A 0.24; carotene 0.12, thiamine 0.02; riboflavin 0.29; nicotinic acid 5.13; folic acid 0.002; vitamin D 0.145µg.

*Cheese spread* contains reduced levels of all vitamins compared with hard cheeses, providing (in mg per 100g): vitamin A 0.18; carotene 0.105; thiamine 0.02; riboflavin 0.24; nicotinic acid 4.37; vitamin D 0.133$\mu$g.

---

**Cheraskin, Emanuel,** American doctor who uses vitamin therapy extensively in treating various diseases, with and without conventional drugs.

---

**cherries,** raw, edible part supplies 120$\mu$g carotene per 100g plus 0.1mg vitamin E. Negligible losses of fat-soluble vitamins when fruit is stewed. B vitamins present are (in mg per 100g), for raw and stewed cherries respectively: thiamine 0.05, 0.03; riboflavin 0.07, 0.06; nicotinic acid 0.4, 0.4; pyridoxine 0.05, 0.02; pantothenic acid 0.4, 0.3. Folic acid reduced from 8 to 3$\mu$g per 100g. Vitamin C content is 5 and 3mg per 100g for raw and stewed cherries respectively.

---

**chestnuts,** edible portion provides a good source of B vitamins and vitamin E. Supplies 7.5mg vitamin E per 100g. B vitamins present are (in mg per 100g): thiamine 0.20; riboflavin 0.22; nicotinic acid 0.6; pyridoxine 0.33; pantothenic acid 0.47. Folic acid level is 1.3$\mu$g per 100g but biotin has not been detected. Traces only of vitamin C present in chestnut kernels. In roasted chestnuts, thiamine level is reduced to 0.04mg per 100g; that of pantothenic acid to 0.08mg per 100g.

---

**chick antidermatitis factor,** *see* pantothenic acid.

---

**chick peas,** Bengal gram type. Moderate source of carotene, vitamin C and B vitamins. Carotene levels for raw and boiled chick peas are respectively (in $\mu$g per 100g) 190, 190. Traces only of vitamin E. Levels of B vitamins for the raw and boiled chick peas are respectively (in mg per 100g): thiamine 0.50, 0.14; riboflavin 0.15, 0.05; nicotinic acid 1.5, 0.5; pyridoxine, not detected; pantothenic acid, not detected. Good source of folic acid at 180 and 37$\mu$g per 100g respectively. Contribute 3mg vitamin C per 100g in raw and boiled states.

---

**chicken,** when cooked supplies only traces of vitamin A, D and carotene. Vitamin E ranges from 0.06 to 0.15 mg per 100g. Concentrations of the B vitamins (in mg per 100g) range from : thiamine 0.05-0.11; riboflavin 0.10-0.28; nicotinic acid 6.4-15.3; pyridoxine 0.13-0.53; pantothenic acid 0.6-1.3; (in μg per 100g) vitamin $B_{12}$ 1.0; biotin 2-4; folic acid 4-13. Completely devoid of vitamin C. *See also* Meats: Cooking losses.

---

**chicory,** in the raw state contains only traces of carotene with no detectable vitamin E. B vitamins present are (in mg per 100g): thiamine 0.05; riboflavin 0.05; nicotinic acid 0.6; pyridoxine 0.05. Reasonable source of folic acid at 52μg per 100g. Vitamin C content is 4mg per 100g.

---

**chilblains,** congestion and swelling of the skin due to cold and attended with severe itching or burning. Can be treated orally with nicotinic acid (25mg) and acetomenaphthone (10mg) per tablet. Complemented by creams containing methylnicotinate (1 per cent) plus other non-vitamin ingredients.

---

**children,** vitamin needs related to weight but requirements for growth must also be accounted for. More likely to have faddy and fickle appetites and have a taste for foods of high calorie intake but low vitamin content. Good diet most important to health but may benefit from low level supplementation of vitamins and minerals. (See Table 2.)

---

**chloramphenicol,** antibiotic. Prevents formation of vitamin K by intestinal bacteria.

---

**chlorbutol,** anti-nausea agent. Enhances excretion and metabolism of vitamin C.

---

**chocolate,** in its various forms, supplies carotene, vitamin E and B vitamins but some of those are supplied by ingredients other than cocoa, e.g. milk. Carotene contents of milk, plain and filled chocolate bars are all 40μg per 100g. Traces only of vitamin D present in milk and filled bars but missing from plain chocolate. Vitamin E levels of milk and plain chocolate bars are 2.9 and 4.0mg per 100g respectively. B vitamins present are (in mg per 100g), for milk, plain and filled chocolate bars respectively: thiamine 0.10, 0.07, 0.10; riboflavin 0.23, 0.08, 0.10; nicotinic acid 1.6, 1.2, 1.0; pyridoxine 0.02, 0.02, 0.02; pantothenic acid 0.6, 0.6, 0.6. Folic acid levels are $10\mu g$ per 100g for all types of chocolate; biotin levels are $3\mu g$ per 100g. Vitamin C is absent.

---

**cholecalciferol,** *see* $D_2$ vitamin.

---

**cholesterol,** fatty substance with three essential functions in the body. Constituent of cell membranes particularly the myelin sheath that insulates nerves; precursor of bile acids; precursor of steroid hormones (sex, anti-stress, water balance, metabolic). Production of steroid hormones needs vitamin C and pantothenic acid.

Cholesterol exists in blood and organs as HDL-cholesterol (high density lipoprotein); LDL-cholesterol (low density lipoprotein); VLDL-cholesterol (very low density lipoprotein). High ratio of HDL to LDL and VLDL desirable to protect against atherosclerosis, arteriosclerosis and coronary heart disease. HDL increased by taking PUFA instead of animal fats; by taking 600IU of vitamin E daily.

*High blood cholesterol* levels reduced by taking 500mg vitamin C daily or by taking 3g nicotinic acid daily.

---

**cholestyramine,** anti-cholesterol agent. Prevents absorption of vitamins A, D, E, K and $B_{12}$.

---

**choline,** water-soluble member of the vitamin B complex. Not regarded as a true vitamin in man since it can be synthesized by the liver. Known also as amanitine, lipotropic factor. Active constituent of lecithin. Present in supplements as choline bitartrate, choline chloride, phosphatidyl choline, lecithin. Colorless, crystalline substance.

*Richest food sources* (in mg per 100g) are desiccated liver (2170); lecithin granules (3430); beef heart (1720); egg-yolk (1700); lecithin oil (800); liver (650); beef steak (600); wheat germ (505); dried brewer's yeast (300); oatflakes (240); nuts (220); legumes (120); corn (100); citrus fruits (85); whole-wheat bread (80); green-leaf vegetables (80); soy flour (70); chicken (60); shellfish (50); bananas (44); root vegetables (40); human milk (35); cow's milk (11).

**Table 2: Recommended dietary intakes for children**

| COUNTRY | AGE (years) | SEX | VIT A µg | VIT D µg | VIT E mg | VIT $B_1$ mg | VIT $B_2$ mg | NICOTINIC ACID mg | VIT $B_6$ mg | FOLIC ACID µg | VIT $B_{12}$ µg | VIT C mg |
|---|---|---|---|---|---|---|---|---|---|---|---|---|
| CANADA | 0-0.5 | Both | 400 | 10 | 3 | 0.3 | 0.4 | 5 | 0.3 | 40 | 0.3 | 20 |
| | 0.5-1.0 | Both | 400 | 10 | 3 | 0.5 | 0.6 | 6 | 0.4 | 60 | 0.3 | 20 |
| | 1-3 | Both | 400 | 10 | 4 | 0.7 | 0.8 | 9 | 0.8 | 100 | 0.4 | 20 |
| | 4-6 | Both | 500 | 5 | 5 | 0.9 | 1.1 | 12 | 1.3 | 100 | 1.5 | 20 |
| | 7-9 | M | 700 | 2.5 | 6 | 1.1 | 1.3 | 14 | 1.6 | 100 | 1.5 | 30 |
| | | F | 700 | 2.5 | 6 | 1.0 | 1.2 | 13 | 1.4 | 100 | 1.5 | 30 |
| | 10-12 | M | 800 | 2.5 | 7 | 1.2 | 1.5 | 17 | 1.8 | 100 | 3.0 | 30 |
| | | F | 800 | 2.5 | 7 | 1.1 | 1.4 | 15 | 1.5 | 100 | 3.0 | 30 |
| | 13-15 | M | 1000 | 2.5 | 9 | 1.4 | 1.7 | 19 | 2.0 | 200 | 3.0 | 30 |
| | | F | 800 | 2.5 | 7 | 1.1 | 1.4 | 15 | 1.5 | 200 | 3.0 | 30 |
| | 16-18 | M | 1000 | 2.5 | 10 | 1.6 | 2.0 | 21 | 2.0 | 200 | 3.0 | 30 |
| | | F | 800 | 2.5 | 6 | 1.1 | 1.3 | 14 | 1.5 | 200 | 3.0 | 30 |
| USA | 0-0.5 | Both | 420 | 10 | 3 | 0.3 | 0.6 | 6 | 0.3 | 30 | 0.5 | 35 |
| | 0.5-1.0 | Both | 400 | 10 | 4 | 0.5 | 0.4 | 8 | 0.6 | 45 | 1.5 | 35 |
| | 1-3 | Both | 400 | 10 | 5 | 0.7 | 0.8 | 9 | 0.9 | 100 | 2.0 | 45 |
| | 4-6 | Both | 500 | 10 | 6 | 0.9 | 1.0 | 11 | 1.3 | 200 | 2.5 | 45 |
| | 7-10 | M | 700 | 10 | 7 | 1.2 | 1.4 | 16 | 1.6 | 300 | 3.0 | 45 |
| | 11-14 | F | 1000 | 10 | 8 | 1.4 | 1.6 | 18 | 1.8 | 400 | 3.0 | 50 |
| | | M | 800 | 10 | 8 | 1.1 | 1.3 | 15 | 1.8 | 400 | 3.0 | 50 |
| | 15-18 | F | 1000 | 10 | 10 | 1.4 | 1.7 | 18 | 2.0 | 400 | 3.0 | 60 |
| | | Both | 800 | 10 | 8 | 1.1 | 1.3 | 14 | 2.0 | 400 | 3.0 | 60 |
| FAO/WHO | 0-1.0 | Both | 300 | 10 | — | 0.3 | 0.5 | 5.4 | — | 60 | 0.3 | 20 |
| | 1-3 | Both | 250 | 10 | — | 0.5 | 0.8 | 9.0 | — | 100 | 0.9 | 20 |
| | 4-6 | Both | 300 | 10 | — | 0.7 | 1.1 | 12.1 | — | 100 | 1.5 | 20 |
| | 7-9 | M | 400 | 2.5 | — | 0.9 | 1.3 | 14.5 | — | 100 | 1.5 | 20 |
| | 10-12 | M | 575 | 2.5 | — | 1.0 | 1.6 | 17.2 | — | 100 | 2.0 | 20 |

| COUNTRY | AGE (years) | SEX | VIT A µg | VIT D µg | VIT E mg | VIT B$_1$ mg | VIT B$_2$ mg | NICOTINIC ACID mg | VIT B$_6$ mg | FOLIC ACID µg ** | VIT B$_{12}$ µg | VIT C mg |
|---|---|---|---|---|---|---|---|---|---|---|---|---|
| FAO/WHO |  | F | 575 | 2.5 | — | 0.9 | 1.4 | 15.5 | — | 100 | 2.0 | 20 |
|  | 13-15 | M | 725 | 2.5 | — | 1.2 | 1.7 | 19.1 | — | 200 | 2.0 | 30 |
|  | 16-19 | F | 725 | 2.5 | — | 1.0 | 1.5 | 16.4 | — | 200 | 2.0 | 30 |
|  |  | M | 750 | 2.5 | — | 1.2 | 1.8 | 20.3 | — | 200 | 2.0 | 30 |
|  |  | F | 750 | 2.5 | — | 0.9 | 1.4 | 15.2 | — | 200 | 2.0 | 30 |
| UK | 0-1 | M | 450 | 7.5 | — | 0.3 | 0.4 | 5 | — | — | — | 20 |
|  |  | F | 450 | 7.5 | — | 0.3 | 0.4 | 5 | — | — | — | 20 |
|  | 1 | M | 300 | 10 | — | 0.5 | 0.6 | 7 | — | — | — | 20 |
|  |  | F | 300 | 10 | — | 0.4 | 0.6 | 7 | — | — | — | 20 |
|  | 2 | M | 300 | 10 | — | 0.6 | 0.7 | 8 | — | — | — | 20 |
|  |  | F | 300 | 10 | — | 0.5 | 0.7 | 8 | — | — | — | 20 |
|  | 3-4 | M | 300 | 10 | — | 0.6 | 0.8 | 9 | — | — | — | 20 |
|  |  | F | 300 | 10 | — | 0.6 | 0.8 | 9 | — | — | — | 20 |
|  | 5-6 | M | 300 | 10* | — | 0.7 | 0.9 | 10 | — | — | — | 20 |
|  |  | F | 300 | 10 | — | 0.7 | 0.9 | 10 | — | — | — | 20 |
|  | 7-8 | M | 400 | 10 | — | 0.8 | 1.0 | 11 | — | — | — | 20 |
|  |  | F | 400 | 10 | — | 0.8 | 1.0 | 11 | — | — | — | 20 |
|  | 9-11 | M | 575 | 10 | — | 0.9 | 1.2 | 14 | — | — | — | 25 |
|  |  | F | 575 | 10 | — | 0.8 | 1.2 | 14 | — | — | — | 25 |
|  | 12-14 | M | 725 | 10 | — | 1.1 | 1.4 | 16 | — | — | — | 25 |
|  |  | F | 725 | 10 | — | 0.9 | 1.4 | 16 | — | — | — | 25 |
|  | 15-17 | M | 750 | 10 | — | 1.2 | 1.7 | 19 | — | — | — | 30 |
|  |  | F | 750 | 10 | — | 0.9 | 1.7 | 19 | — | — | — | 30 |

* Supplements of 10µg daily recommended only during winter months for children and adolescents of more than 5 years of age.
** Folic acid intakes not yet recommended.

45

*Stable* to cooking methods and food processing.

*Absorbed* better as phosphatidyl choline and lecithin than as choline bitartrate and choline chloride.

*Functions* as precursor of betaine, important in body metabolic reactions; as acetylcholine, essential for nerve impulse transmission; as lipotropic factor that prevents accumulation of fats in liver and other organs; as stimulator of phospholipid production, essential component of cell membranes.

*Deficiency in man* causes no specific disease but may give rise to fatty liver, nerve degeneration, high blood pressure, lack of resistance to infection, reduced immunity system; atherosclerosis; thrombosis; stroke; high blood cholesterol.

*Deficiency symptoms* are those associated with above conditions but may not be specific for choline deficiency alone.

*Deficiency in animals* leads to fatty liver followed by cirrhosis; hemorrhage of liver, kidney, lungs; defective leg joints (turkeys).

*Recommended dietary intakes* have not been set by any authority. Normal daily intake on good mixed diet calculated at between 300 and 1000mg.

*Increased intakes* required by diabetics; alcohol drinkers.

*Toxicity* of choline as bitartrate and chloride is low but as phosphatidyl choline and lecithin is even lower. No serious side-effects even at high doses.

*Therapy* with choline beneficial in atherosclerosis; angina; thrombosis; stroke; high blood pressure; senile dementia; Alzheimer's disease.

---

**cider,**  all kinds provide fewer B vitamins than beers and lagers. Traces only of carotene. B vitamins present are (in mg per 100ml): thiamine, trace; riboflavin, trace; nicotinic acid 0.01; pyridoxine 0.005; pantothenic acid 0.03. Biotin level is 1µg per 100ml; folic acid has not been measured. All ciders are devoid of vitamin C.

---

**cigarette smoking,**  four main poisons are acetaldehyde, cancer-producing substances (carcinogens), carbon monoxide and nicotine.

Toxic effects of acetaldehyde, carbon monoxide and nicotine neutralized by vitamin $B_1$, vitamin C and cysteine. Beta-carotene protects against carcinogens.

Heavy smoking can inactivate vitamin $B_{12}$, inducing pernicious anemia and eventually blindness. Treat with injections of hydroxocobalamin.

---

**cirrhosis,** chronic, progressive disease of the liver characterized by destruction of liver cells and overgrowth of connective tissue. Complementary vitamin treatment includes high doses of vitamin B complex plus fat-soluble vitamins A, D, E and K to overcome excessive loss due to disease. Choline (up to 3000mg daily) may be needed to prevent fatty infiltration.

---

**citrovorum factor,** *see* folinic acid.

---

**claudication,** intermittent. Pains in calves induced by walking and due to narrowing of leg blood vessels. Treated with vitamin E, 400-600IU daily.

---

**cobalamin,** *see* $B_{12}$ vitamin.

---

**cocoa,** the powder supplies carotene, vitamin E and some B vitamins but is devoid of vitamin C. Carotene level is 40μg per 100g. Vitamin E content is 3.2mg per 100g. B vitamins present are (in mg per 100g): thiamine 0.16; riboflavin 0.06; nicotinic acid 7.3; pyridoxine 0.07. Folic acid level is 38μg per 100g.

---

**coconut,** supplies less vitamin E and B vitamins than other nuts but does contain some vitamin C. Desiccated coconut is richer in most vitamins than fresh edible portion. Vitamin E level of edible portion is 1.0mg per 100g; desiccated variety is devoid of vitamin E. B vitamins present are (in mg per 100g) for fresh and desiccated coconut respectively: thiamine 0.03, 0.06; riboflavin 0.02, 0.04; nicotinic acid 1.0, 1.8; pyridoxine 0.04, 0.09; pantothenic acid 0.20, 0.31. Folic acid levels are 26 and 54μg per 100g respectively for fresh and desiccated coconut. Vitamin C content of fresh coconut is 2mg per 100g but there is none in the desiccated variety.

*Coconut milk* supplies traces of most vitamins that are in the flesh. Traces only of vitamin E. B vitamins present are (in mg per 100g): thiamine, and riboflavin, traces only; nicotinic acid 0.2; pyridoxine 0.03; pantothenic acid 0.05. No folic acid or biotin have been detected. Vitamin C level is 2mg per 100g.

---

**cod-liver oil,** rich source of fat-soluble vitamins but completely devoid of water-soluble variety. Provides (in mg per 100g): vitamin A 18.0; vitamin D 0.21; vitamin E 20.0.

Contains also polyunsaturated fatty acids known as Eicosapentenoic Acid (EPA) 9.0 per cent and Docosahexenoic Acid (DHA) 8.0 per cent that have essential roles in body metabolism. Total polyunsaturated fatty acids (vitamin F) present at level of 23g per 100g oil.

---

**coffee,** all types of coffee are devoid of carotene and vitamin E. Rich source of nicotinic acid.

*Ground, roasted variety* supplies 0.20mg riboflavin per 100g and 10.0mg nicotinic acid per 100g. The quantity of nicotinic acid increases during the roasting process because it is liberated from a bound form. A dark roasted variety may contain 30 to 40mg nicotinic acid per 100g. No other vitamins have been measured.

*Infused ground coffee* supplies much lower quantities of the above vitamins. Riboflavin content is 0.01mg per 100g. Nicotinic acid content is 0.7mg per 100g.

*Instant coffee* (in dried form) is a very rich source of nicotinic acid at between 24.9 and 41.5mg per 100g. Riboflavin content is 0.11mg per 100g. Also contains pyridoxine (0.03mg per 100g) and pantothenic acid (0.4mg per 100g).

*Decaffeinated coffee* (in dried form) provides similar vitamin levels to ground, roasted variety. Instant decaffeinated coffee has similar vitamin levels to instant coffee.

---

**coffee and chicory extract,** very few vitamins have been measured. Riboflavin content is 0.03mg per 100g; nicotinic acid content is 2.8mg per 100g.

---

**colchicine,** used to treat gout. Prevents absorption of vitamins A and $B_{12}$.

---

**cold,** viral infection of the upper respiratory tract. Also known as coryza, rhinitis, head cold.

Increase vitamin A intake during period of illness. Treat with vitamin C at intake of 1 gram every 4 hours until relief obtained, then gradually reduce over one week to 1 gram per day then 500mg maintenance dose.

**colitis,** chronic, inflammatory and ulcerative disease of the colon. Drug treatment should be supplemented with high potency multivitamin preparation plus extra vitamin C and $B_6$ when on corticosteroids.

**collagen,** main protein of connective tissues (skin, joints, vital organs) throughout body. Starting material for production of gelatin. Rate of wound healing depends upon rate of production of collagen, itself dependent on vitamin C.

Vitamin C (500 to 1000mg daily) often given routinely to patients undergoing surgery and those recovering from accidental injury to accelerate healing process.

**colon cancer,** *see* cancer.

**compound cooking fat,** apart from trace of vitamin E, completely devoid of all vitamins.

**confections,** boiled sweets, fruit gums, liquorice products, pastilles, peppermints and toffee are generally devoid of all vitamins. Some nicotinic acid in liquorice (0.7mg per 100g) and in milk toffee (0.4mg per 100g), but this vitamin is supplied by the liquorice root and the milk ingredient respectively. *See also* Chocolate.

**constipation,** stubborn cases may respond to vitamin $B_1$ (10mg daily). Complete vitamin B complex sometimes used to stimulate intestinal bacteria growth to relieve constipation, particularly after antibiotic treatment.

**contraceptives,** *IUD (intra-uterine device).* Excessive bleeding controlled by bioflavonoids (1000mg daily) *or* vitamin E (100IU every other day).

*Oral.* Consist of synthetic estrogens and progestogens that can increase requirements for certain vitamins. Supplementary vitamin $B_6$ (25-50mg), vitamin $B_{12}$ (5µg), folic acid (200µg), vitamin E (100IU) and vitamin C (100mg) needed daily.

*Barrier* types, such as condom or diaphragm, with or without contraceptive creams or jellies, have no known effect on vitamin requirements.

---

**convalescence,** stage of post-illness often characterized by mild deficiency of vitamins induced by low food intake and by medicinal drugs. Supplement with all-round multivitamin preparation plus extra vitamin C (500-1000mg) in illnesses of infection and in post-operative period.

---

**cooking losses in vegetables,** losses depend upon: (a) volume of water used; (b) time of cooking, and (c) extent of chopping of vegetables. Percentage losses of vitamins are given in Table 3. Highest losses are associated with large volume of cooking water, long time boiling and finely divided vegetables.

**Table 3: Percentage losses of vitamins in the cooking process**

|  | *Root vegetables* | *Leafy vegetables* | *Seeds* |
|---|---|---|---|
| Carotene | 0 | 0 | 0 |
| Thiamine | 25 | 40 | 30 |
| Riboflavin | 30 | 40 | 30 |
| Nicotinic acid | 30 | 40 | 30 |
| Pyridoxine | 40 | 40 | 40 |
| Pantothenic acid | 30 | 30 | 30 |
| Folic acid | 50 | 30 | 50 |
| Biotin | 30 | 30 | 30 |
| Vitamin E | 0 | 0 | 0 |
| Vitamin C | 40 | 70 | 60 |

---

**corn,** in the raw state is good source of carotene and all vitamins. Water-soluble vitamins are lost when boiled and when canned. The raw, boiled and canned kernels contain 240, 240 and 210µg carotene per 100g respectively. Similarly vitamin E levels are 2.4, 1.5 and 1.5mg per 100g respectively. Boiling reduces concentrations of the B vitamins which are further reduced by canning. These are (in mg per 100g), for raw, boiled and canned respectively: thiamine 0.20, 0.15, 0.05; riboflavin 0.08, 0.08, 0.08; nicotinic acid 2.2, 2.1, 1.5; pyridoxine 0.19, 0.16, 0.16; pantothenic acid 0.54, 0.38, 0.22. Folic acid levels are also reduced accordingly to give contents of 52, 33, and 32$\mu$g per 100g respectively. Biotin appears to be absent.

**cornstarch,** the starch granules of corn. Completely devoid of carotene, vitamin E and vitamin C. Traces only of thiamine, riboflavin, nicotinic acid, pyridoxine, pantothenic acid, folic acid and biotin.

**cortocosteroids,** hormones produced by the adrenal glands from cholesterol. These plus synthetic analogues (called steroid drugs) used extensively in medicine at relatively high levels. Adversely affect certain vitamins. Increase requirements of vitamins $B_6$ and C and probably D. Needs are $B_6$ (25-50mg daily in both sexes), C (500-1000mg daily) and D (400IU daily).

**cortisol,** a natural corticosteroid. *See* corticosteroids.

**cortisone,** a natural corticosteroid. *See* corticosteroids.

**coryza,** head cold. *See* cold.

**co-trimoxazole,** antibacterial agent. Impairs folic acid utilization.

**Cott, Allan,** American doctor who pioneered megavitamin therapy for emotional disorders with particular reference to learning disabilities in children.

**cramps,** leg. When induced by exercise is called intermittent claudication. Nocturnal (night-time) cramps treated with vitamin E (200IU daytime, 200IU before sleep) plus vitamin C (500mg daily). Cramps due to restless leg syndrome treated with vitamin E (400IU daily).

---

**cranberries,** when raw provide 20µg carotene per 100g; negligible vitamin E. B vitamins present are (in mg per 100g): thiamine 0.03; riboflavin 0.06; nicotinic acid 0.4; pyridoxine 0.04; pantothenic acid 0.22. Supply only 2µg per 100g folic acid; no detectable biotin. Useful source of vitamin C at 12mg per 100g.

---

**cream,** shows seasonal variations in fat-soluble vitamins. Water-soluble constant levels are (in mg per 100g): thiamine 0.03; riboflavin 0.12; nicotinic acid 0.64; pyridoxine 0.03; folic acid 0.004; pantothenic acid 0.30; biotin 0.0014; vitamin C 1.2; vitamin $B_{12}$ 0.2µg.

*Summer light cream* provides (per 100g): vitamin A 0.2mg; carotene 0.125mg; vitamin E 0.5mg; vitamin D 0.165µg. *Winter light cream* provides (per 100g): vitamin A 0.145mg; carotene 0.07mg; vitamin E 0.4mg; vitamin D 0.081µg. *Heavy cream* contains approximately twice the quantity of fat-soluble vitamins as light cream.

---

**Crohn's disease,** generalized inflammatory disease of the small intestine and lower intestinal tract. Also known as regional enteritis. Drug treatment complemented by high potency multivitamin supplementation. Extra vitamin C and $B_6$ also recommended when on corticosteroids.

---

**cucumber,** traces only of carotene and vitamin E. Levels of B vitamins (in mg per 100g) are: thiamine 0.04; riboflavin 0.04; nicotinic acid 0.3; pyridoxine 0.04; pantothenic acid 0.30. Contributes 16µg folic acid per 100g but traces only of biotin. Vitamin C content is 8mg per 100g.

---

**currants,** *see* dried currants and specific types.

---

**cyanocobalamin,** *see* $B_{12}$ vitamin.

---

**cycloserine,** antibiotic. Reduces availability of folic acid.

---

**cystic fibrosis,** inherited disease usually starting in infancy and typified by chronic infection of respiratory system, pancreatic insufficiency and susceptibility to heat. Infection needs increased vitamin C intake (up to 1000mg daily); pancreatic insufficiency leads to fat malabsorption so increased intakes of vitamin A (7500IU), vitamin D (400IU), vitamin E (250IU) needed daily.

---

**cysts,** cystic disease of the breast, a benign condition, is the most common disease of the female breast, occurring in about 5 per cent of middle-aged women. Pain or premenstrual breast discomfort is a frequent symptom and cyst may be tender but more often condition has no symptoms. Discovery usually by palpation.

Once malignancy has been discounted, treatment, apart from surgery, may be two-fold:

1. 600IU vitamin E daily for eight weeks should give clinical response;

2. oil of evening primrose, 3000mg daily divided into three doses.

---

# D

---

**D,** fat-soluble vitamin. Occurs naturally as cholecalciferol ($D_2$) found only in animal sources and ergocalciferol ($D_2$) produced by the action of light on yeast. Isolated in 1930 from cod liver oil by Dr. E. Mallanby. One microgram is equivalent to 40 international units.

*Richest sources* are (in mcg per 100g) cod-liver oil (210); kippers (25.0); mackerel (17.5); canned salmon (12.5); sardines (7.5) and tuna (5.8). Dairy products include eggs (highest at 1.75); cow's milk (lowest at 0.03). Added to margarine to give $8\mu g/100g$.

Usually incorporated into supplements as ergocalciferol but sometimes as cod liver oil. Stable to most cooking and food processing techniques. Significant amounts of cholecalciferol are produced by the action of sunlight on 7-dehydrocholesterol in the skin. Vitamin D functions only after conversion to 25-hydroxy vitamin D by the liver and further conversion to 1,25-dihydroxy vitamin D by the kidneys.

*Functions* of these compounds are:

1. to promote absorption of calcium from the small intestine;
2. to promote absorption of phosphate from the small intestine;
3. to cause release of calcium from bone.

*Deficiency* leads to rickets in children and osteomalacia in adults, both diseases characterized by softening of the bones due to lack of calcium phosphate.

*Deficiency symptoms* in rickets include unnatural limb posture, excessive sweating of the head, delayed ability to stand, sit up, crawl and walk. Knock-knees or bow legs develop once the child can stand. In osteomalacia bone pain is present in the ribs, lower spine, pelvis and legs. Muscular weakness and spasms are common. Bones become brittle and easily broken.

*Deficiency in animals* causes inhibition of growth, accelerated respiration (calf), muscle cramp (pig), bowed legs, enlarged joints (cows), thin shelled eggs (poultry) and infertility, deformed young at birth.

*Recommended daily intakes* in the USA and Europe are 10µg (400IU) throughout life. In the UK intakes are 10µg (400IU) up to 7 years of age then 2.5µg (100IU) from then on. Should be increased to 10µg during pregnancy and breast-feeding.

*Highest supplementary intake* permitted is 10µg daily in both the USA and UK in medicines available without prescription.

Most toxic of all the vitamins. *Toxicity symptoms* in infants include loss of appetite, nausea, vomiting, constant thirst and head pains. The child becomes thin, irritable and depressed. Calcium is deposited in the organs and soft tissues of the body culminating in obvious growths. Similar symptoms seen in adults.

*Therapy* with vitamin D essential in rickets and osteomalacia. Has been used to treat osteoporosis and rheumatoid arthritis.

---

**Dam H.,** Danish scientist who first demonstrated disease due to deficiency of vitamin K (1934), then isolated the vitamin from alfalfa and decayed fish meal (1935). Nobel Prize winner.

---

**damsons,** variety of plums. Useful source of carotene and vitamin E but little vitamin C present. Stewing the fruit reduces potency of B vitamins, due mainly to dilution with water and losses into water. Carotene contents (in $\mu$g per 100g) for raw (edible part only), stewed without sugar and stewed with sugar are respectively 220, 180, 170; vitamin E levels (in mg per 100g) are respectively 0.7, 0.6 and 0.5. B vitamins present (in mg per 100g) for raw (edible part only), stewed without sugar and stewed with sugar are respectively: thiamine 0.10, 0.08, 0.06; riboflavin 0.03, 0.03, 0.02; nicotinic acid 0.4, 0.4, 0.3; pyridoxine 0.05, 0.03, 0.03; pantothenic acid 0.27, 0.21, 0.18. Traces only of folic acid (3, 1 and 1$\mu$g respectively) and biotin (stable at 0.1$\mu$g). Vitamin C is only 3, 3 and 2mg per 100g respectively.

---

**dates,** when dried, edible part supplies carotene and B vitamins. Supplies 50$\mu$g carotene per 100g; but no measurable vitamin E. B vitamins present (in mg per 100g) are: thiamine 0.07; riboflavin 0.04; nicotinic acid 2.9; pyridoxine 0.15; pantothenic acid 0.80. Folic acid level is 21$\mu$g per 100g but biotin is absent. No vitamin C present.

---

**deafness,** may be due to otosclerosis, a disease where the bones of the middle ear become fused, unable to vibrate and transmit sound. Particularly in elderly where it may be related to long-term vitamin A deficiency. Cannot be cured by vitamin therapy but adequate intakes throughout life may prevent it.

---

**decubitus ulcer,** *see* bedsores.

---

**deficiency,** lack of sufficient vitamin intake. For example, four stages of vitamin deficiency identified in volunteers deprived of B$_1$:

1. no obvious changes in first 5-10 days but vitamin stores depleted;
2. altered cell metabolism after 10-60 days;
3. clinical defects after 30-180 days with non-specific symptoms like weight loss, appetite loss, malaise, insomnia, increased irritability;
4. anatomical defects from 180 days on leading to specific signs of gross deficiency that if untreated may lead to death.

Can be caused by poor nutrition; poor cooking methods; overprocessing and over-refining of foods; habits like smoking tobacco and drinking alcohol; stress; medicinal drugs; contraceptive pill; malabsorption; inefficient utilization.

---

**deficiency causes,** there are many factors that can give rise to mild vitamin deficiency and most individuals are prone to the influence of one or more.

*Apathy* — is often a feature of people living alone, particularly those who have lost a spouse and those who no longer have a family to look after. There is little incentive to prepare adequate meals. Meals are often monotonous and less and less nourishing. Impaired digestion may be associated with the apathy and this further lowers the nutritional status. Often seen in the elderly, middle-aged bachelor or spinster living in a one-room apartment with poor cooking facilities or in teenagers and students living alone for the first time.

*Dental problems* — poor dentition due to loss of teeth or dental decay can make eating uncomfortable, leading to aversion to foods such as salads, meat and vegetables. An ill-balanced diet results, which can lead to poor nutrition, particularly in the elderly.

*Excessive losses* — water-soluble vitamins tend to be excreted in the urine and sweat. Physical exertion can thus lead to excessive excretion of vitamins. Hot climates may have a similar effect.

*Food fads* — deficiencies often occur in the young when foods of high calorie intake but low vitamin content are popular and make up the main part of the diet, e.g. high-sugar foods, soft drinks, confections, potato snacks, sweets, cakes. Old people too are not immune from similar nutritional fads. Food fads of pregnancy are well known and very variable but it has been suggested they may be satisfying a demand by the woman for specific nutrients.

*Food taboos* — often are religious in origin but may also stem from public health ideas, e.g. avoiding meat prone to parasitic infection. Complete avoidance of food as in fasting may be beneficial as an occasional habit but extensive fasting can be harmful. Water-soluble vitamins may be depleted and body protein is known to be broken down as well as body fat.

Specific foods that are nutritionally sound are avoided because of superstitious belief, completely unfounded, that they do harm. Many such beliefs abound in Africa. In Bolivia, any food containing animal blood is believed to make children mute; in Pakistan buffalo milk is believed to make a person physically strong but mentally dull. Most affected are pregnant women who often suffer nutritionally from such beliefs at a period when their diet should be sound. Sometimes because they are pregnant they are denied certain foods acceptable to them in other circumstances, so they suffer twice over.

*Individual requirements* — minimum daily requirements of vitamins are based on average intakes of a population or are an extension of animal studies applied to humans. Experiments indicate that animals of the same species can vary one from another in their vitamin requirements as much as five-fold. It is likely that human beings vary also so that two people on a similar diet can show wide variation in blood levels of vitamins which may also reflect requirements.

*Infections* — are more likely in those suffering from malnutrition, particularly among children. Infections can also aggravate malnutrition (e.g. by reducing the appetite) and in turn malnutrition weakens resistance to infection. Infections most likely to occur in malnourished children are bacterial (e.g. tuberculosis), viral (measles, which can be a killing disease in malnutrition) and parasitic. Deficiencies of vitamins A and C are most likely to predispose to infections. Keratomalacia, the end stage of vitamin A deficiency resulting in blindness, is often aggravated by a concurrent infection in children. Vitamin deficiency may lower resistance to infection by a reduced antibody formation; reduced activity of bacterial- and viral-engulfing white blood cells (phagocytes); decreased levels of protective enzymes (e.g. lysozyme in tears) and reduced integrity of the skin and mucous membranes, the wet surfaces of the body.

Infections can precipitate gross deficiencies of vitamins in those on a poor diet and even mild deficiencies in those on an adequate diet. For example, children with meningococcal meningitis, diarrhea, tuberculosis, measles and other acute infections can develop vitamin A deficiency severe enough to cause them to develop keratomalacia and eventually blindness. Fever can cause symptoms of scurvy, due to vitamin C deficiency, in children even when there are apparently adequate intakes of the vitamin. Gross signs of thiamine deficiency can be precipitated in borderline cases following infections; diarrhea and beriberi results.

*Lactation* — little is known about precise vitamin requirements in the woman who is breast-feeding her child and ignorance is reflected in the varying figures suggested by different authorities. All agree, however, that increased vitamin intakes during this period are desirable.

Suggested vitamin intakes are given in Table 4.

# D | THE DICTIONARY OF VITAMINS

**Table 4: Suggested vitamin intakes during lactation**

|  | Australia | Canada | New Zealand | UK | USA | WHO/FAO |
|---|---|---|---|---|---|---|
| Vitamin A μg | 1200 | 1400 | 1200 | 750 | 1200 | 1200 |
| Vitamin D μg | 10 | 5.0 | 10 | 10 | 10 | 10 |
| Vitamin E mg | — | 8.0 | 13.5 | — | 11 | — |
| Vitamin C mg | 60 | 60 | 60 | 60 | 100 | 60 |
| Thiamine mg | 1.3 | 1.5 | 1.3 | 1.1 | 1.6 | 1.1 |
| Riboflavin mg | 1.7 | 1.7 | 2.5 | 1.8 | 1.7 | 1.7 |
| Nicotinic acid mg | 22 | 25 | 21 | 21 | 18 | 18.2 |
| Pyridoxine mg | 3.5 | 2.6 | 2.5 | — | 2.5 | — |
| Folic acid μg | 300 | 250 | 400 | — | 500 | 500 |
| Vitamin B$_{12}$ μg | 2.5 | 3.5 | 4.0 | — | 4.0 | 4.5 |

*Malabsorption* — usually affects the fat-soluble vitamins but pernicious anemia is due solely to an inability to absorb the water-soluble vitamin B$_{12}$.

Diseases such as sprue, idiopathic steatorrhea, pancreatic diseases, lack of bile production, etc., can cause generalized malabsorption of fats which include the fat-soluble vitamins and so can give rise to deficiency. Lack of intrinsic factor, needed to complex with vitamin B$_{12}$ as a prerequisite for absorption, prevents the assimilation of the vitamin.

Malabsorption problems are medical conditions that are the province of the medical doctor and unsuitable for self-treatment.

*Medicinal drugs* — most common vitamin deficiency is that of B complex during antibiotic therapy. Essential to supplement with whole of vitamin B complex for any antibiotic taken for more than three days. Pyridoxine is particularly vulnerable during drug therapy but especially with corticosteroids, oral contraceptives, isoniazid and penicillamine. *See* individual drugs.

*Other food nutrients* — may affect the needs for certain vitamins. For example, high polyunsaturated fatty acid intake (as in vegetable oils) requires high vitamin E levels to accompany it; thiamine intake is increased when high carbohydrate levels are part of the diet; high protein intake requires more pyridoxine to be taken at the same time, as well as extra riboflavin. Less of this vitamin is retained when protein intake is low.

Leucine is an amino acid that in high concentration requires extra nicotinic acid. Millet is a food with high leucine content and is a significant part of the diet in India but nicotinic acid intake does not always parallel that of the need, and deficiency of the vitamin can be induced.

Avidin is a protein unique to raw egg-white that combines with and

58

inactivates biotin. Cooking the egg-white destroys avidin and so prevents the inactivation of the vitamin.

Some raw fish contain an enzyme thiaminase that destroys thiamine. Where raw fish is part of the staple diet, as in the Far East, thiamine deficiency can be induced. Some bacteria, e.g. Bacillus thiaminolyticus, can break down thiamine. Some 3 per cent of Japanese are afflicted with this infective organism and show signs of mild thiamine deficiency.

*Other vitamins* — excessive intakes of one vitamin may induce deficiency of another. Occurs mainly in animal experimentation but one established case in humans is where an excess of folic acid can cause a deficiency of vitamin $B_{12}$. In lambs, rickets can be induced in animals with a just-adequate intake of vitamin D by feeding high levels of carotene.

A deficiency of one vitamin can also induce a deficiency of another, e.g. vitamin C is needed to convert folic acid to its active form folinic acid. In the absence of vitamin C, folic acid cannot be activated and anemia results. High intakes of folic acid in humans can mask a deficiency of vitamin $B_{12}$. Lack of folic acid gives rise to an anemia similar to that caused by lack of vitamin $B_{12}$. However, vitamin $B_{12}$ deficiency also causes nerve degeneration in the spinal column. If only the anemia is being monitored, treatment with folic acid of $B_{12}$ deficiency may appear to cure the anemia. The nerve degeneration is not affected and progresses until it becomes irreversible. Hence the importance of diagnosing whether anemia is due to folic acid or vitamin $B_{12}$ deficiency, because the two vitamins function together in the production of normal red blood cells.

*Parasitic infections* — produce specifically vitamin $B_{12}$ deficiency. The parasite responsible is fish tape-worm which utilizes dietary vitamin $B_{12}$, making it unavailable for absorption.

*Physical activity* — increases the need for certain vitamins, particularly those concerned with stress (the vitamin B complex), energy requirements (thiamine) and muscle action (vitamins C and E). If increased levels are not supplied, mild deficiency can result. Recommended dietary allowances for men (20 to 26 years) in three different countries are given in Table 5. *See also* Athletes.

**Table 5: Recommended vitamin requirements for men aged 20-26 years.**

|  |  | UK | West Germany | USSR |
|---|---|---|---|---|
| Thiamine mg | Sedentary | 1.0 | 1.7 | 1.8 |
|  | Moderately active | 1.2 | 2.2 | 2.0 |
|  | Active | 1.4 | 2.5 | 2.5 |
|  | Very active | 1.7 | 2.9 | 3.0 |

|  |  | UK | West Germany | USSR |
|---|---|---|---|---|
| Riboflavin mg | Sedentary | 1.5 | 1.8 | 2.0 |
| | Moderately active | 1.8 | 1.8 | 2.5 |
| | Active | 2.1 | 1.8 | 3.0 |
| | Very active | 2.6 | 1.8 | 3.5 |
| Nicotinic acid mg | Sedentary | 8 | 14 | 12 |
| | Moderately active | 8 | 16 | 15 |
| | Active | 8 | 18 | 20 |
| | Very active | 8 | 20 | 25 |
| Vitamin C mg | Sedentary | 30 | 75 | 60 |
| | Moderately active | 30 | 75 | 70 |
| | Active | 30 | 75 | 100 |
| | Very active | 30 | 75 | 120 |

*Poor diet* — a poor selection of foods coupled with bad cooking methods, over-processing and over-refining can give rise to deficiency of vitamins. *See* Losses in food processing.

*Poor digestion* — can be caused by defective mastication of the food in the mouth; reduction of volume and acidity of gastric secretions; reduction of digestive enzymes in pancreatic, liver and intestinal secretions and reduction of bile secretion. Vitamins are liberated as food is digested so when this is inefficient, they do not become available for absorption.

*Pregnancy* — many studies indicate marked reductions in blood levels of vitamin A, nicotinic acid, pyridoxine, vitamin $B_{12}$, folic acid and vitamin C in pregnant women.

Most comprehensive studies were on pyridoxine and it has been concluded that pregnant women need 10mg of the vitamin daily to maintain normal metabolic functions compared with only 2mg in non-pregnant women.

Folic acid is the most common deficiency. Recommended intakes during pregnancy are given in Table 6.

**Table 6: Recommended vitamin requirements during pregnancy.**

|  | Australia | Canada | New Zealand | UK | USA | WHO/ FAO |
|---|---|---|---|---|---|---|
| Vitamin A μg | 750 | 900 | 750 | 750 | 1000 | 750 |
| Vitamin D μg | 10 | 5.0 | 10 | 10 | 10 | 10 |
| Vitamin E mg | — | 7.0 | 13.5 | — | 10 | — |
| Vitamin C mg | 60 | 50 | 60 | 60 | 80 | 60 |
| Thiamine mg | 1.2 | 1.2 | 1.2 | 1.0 | 1.4 | 1.0 |
| Riboflavin mg | 1.5 | 1.5 | 2.5 | 1.6 | 1.5 | 1.5 |
| Nicotinic acid mg | 19 | 15 | 21 | 18 | 15 | 16.8 |
| Pyridoxine mg | 2.6 | 2.0 | 2.5 | — | 2.6 | — |
| Folic acid μg | 400 | 250 | 500 | — | 800 | 600 |
| Vitamin B$_{12}$ μg | 3.0 | 4.0 | 4.0 | — | 4.0 | 5.0 |

*Rapid growth* — the growing child needs vitamins for the growth process as well as for normal metabolism. Most studies have been carried out in animal husbandry when it was established that optimum levels of vitamins rather than adequate intakes were required to ensure maximum growth. However, most authorities agree that the need in children is relatively higher than that in adults when worked out on a body-weight or food-intake basis.

*Slimming diets* — when undertaken without professional advice, reduced food and calorie intake may not supply the minimum requirements of vitamins. These are required for health irrespective of calories in the diet, apart perhaps from thiamine. A reduction of calories from 2500 to 1000 per day which most slimming diets supply is hence likely also to reduce the vitamin intake by a similar factor. If 2500 calories are supplying barely the minimum needs of vitamins, deficiency must result if calories are reduced to 1000. All slimming regimes should include a good all-round multivitamin-multimineral preparation daily as insurance against deficiency. This may also prevent the tiredness often associated with slimming diets.

*Stress* — any stressful situation increases the requirements of some vitamins, notably the B group, C and E. If increased amounts are not taken in the diet mild deficiency may result. Quantities required may be 2, 3 or even 5 times the normal intakes. *See also* Stress; Athletes.

---

**deficiency groups,** it is now recognized by some authorities (including the UK) that certain sectors of the population may be at risk of being deficient in vitamins and minerals and would benefit from supplementation. In most cases, a general all-round multivitamin-multimineral preparation supplying the minimum daily requirements is sufficient when taken regularly. For the reasons for lowered intake in these groups, *see* deficiency causes.

Groups at risk of deficiency are:

1.  pregnant women, *see* deficiency causes: Pregnancy.
2.  nursing mothers, *see* deficiency causes: Lactation.
3.  women of child-bearing age who may need supplementary iron. Simultaneous supplementation with vitamin C will ensure efficient absorption of the mineral in the proportion 100mg vitamin to 10mg iron.
4.  those who embark on a weight-reducing diet without professional advice. *See* deficiency causes: Slimming diets.
5.  those who eat nutritionally inadequate snacks or foods which may have been overcooked or kept for long periods, thus losing most of their content of the more labile vitamins. *See* deficiency causes: Poor diet.
6.  Children and adolescents in winter and housebound adults who may not get sufficient vitamin D from sunlight falling on the skin. In the absence of sufficient dietary vitamin D, that produced in the skin becomes the main source of supply of the vitamin.
7.  children and adolescents who, because of fads, do not have a properly balanced diet. *See* deficiency causes: Food fads.
8.  those convalescing from an illness who have leeway to make up in their nutrition. Deficiency of vitamins in convalescents is caused by: (a) low intake of food during illness; (b) effect of medicinal drugs; (c) infection, if it is present. *See* deficiency causes: Infections; Medicinal drugs.
9.  the elderly and others who, through varied disabilities or apathy, fail to prepare balanced meals. *See* deficiency causes: Apathy; Dental problems; Poor digestion.
10.  those who live alone and often do not trouble to prepare fresh or adequate meals.
11.  athletes in training and those in physically active occupations. *See* athletes; deficiency causes: Physical activity.

---

**deficiency symptoms,**  specific symptoms and signs exist for most of the vitamin deficiencies, particularly when the vitamin level is seriously reduced and at this stage is the province of the medical practitioner. However, mild abnormalities that could be associated with a less serious deficiency of a vitamin are now being recognized in certain sectors of the population. In this respect, certain areas of the body provide useful information and, with proper interpretation, coupled usually with physical examination and medical history, can indicate poor nutrition. The more obvious areas are the skin, the mouth and the eyes but some symptoms of the gastro-intestinal tract and the nerves can become apparent to the individual affected. Changes in the blood, the blood vessels, the heart, the bones and the reproductive system associated with vitamin deficiency require more sophisticated diagnostic techniques that are best left to the medical practitioner.

*The skin* — much of what is known about the effects of vitamin deficiencies has come from animal studies and these do not always translate to the human being, but skin problems can often respond to vitamin A.

Vitamin A — hard, stippled skin, known as toad skin, has been attributed to vitamin deficiency but it may also be attributed in part to polyunsaturated fatty acid deficiency. Small, raised lesions that are hard and deeply pigmented have been suggested as due to vitamin A deficiency. Many minor skin irritations and those like eczema, acne and psoriasis often respond to vitamin A treatment, both topical and oral, which suggest that they are due, at least in part, to vitamin A deficiency.

Vitamin E — wounds that fail to heal or scar tissue that is consistently painful or striae that will not disappear may be associated with vitamin E deficiency.

Vitamin K — purple patches under the skin (known as purpura) may reflect a prothrombin deficiency which in turn may result from lack of vitamin K.

Vitamin C — small effusions of blood beneath the skin, known as petechiae, scattered in a diffuse manner over various skin areas are characteristic of vitamin C deficiency. Hardened pimples that appear over hair follicles particularly on the calves and buttocks may indicate vitamin C deficiency. The hairs either fail to erupt or take on a spiral shape.

Pyridoxine — deficiency causes scaly, dry skin and excessive looseness and hence loss of body hair. Excessive secretion of the sebaceous glands, known as seborrhea, is seen about the eyes, nose, lips and mouth, sometimes extending to the eyebrows and ears. Redness of the moist surfaces of the body is also a sign of pyridoxine deficiency. Scaly, pigmented dermatitis sometimes occurs around the neck, forearms, elbows and thigh.

Riboflavin — typical skin lesions include cracking of the lips and angles of the mouth, known as cheilosis; seborrhea of the nose and lips; scrotal and vaginal dermatitis; mouth and tongue ulcers.

Nicotinic acid — gross deficiency causes pellagra where the initial change is a temporary redness like sunburn. This clears to produce a more severe coloration in the form of deep red spots that coalesce to form a dark red or purple eruption followed by scaling and loss of skin. Face, neck, hands and feet are most affected, sometimes with concomitant edema and ulceration. Usually clearly defined rough patches on hand termed "pellagrous glove."

Pantothenic acid — in animals, deficiency symptoms are greying of hair and ulceration of the skin but no evidence that human beings show similar signs. "Burning feet" syndrome on soles of feet may be nervous rather than skin deficiency symptom. Some skin lesions like those noted with riboflavin deficiency have responded to pantothenic acid therapy suggesting they are more likely due to multivitamin lack.

Biotin — a localized, scaly, shedding dermatitis is a symptom of deficiency in infants.

*The mouth* — lesions of the mouth include those of the lips and are accepted as specific in some cases for certain deficiencies.

Riboflavin — a sore tongue with cracking of the lips and angles of the mouth, sometimes accompanied by intractable mouth ulceration are features of deficiency. The tongue is magenta-colored with deep fissures and raised pimples (papillae).

Nicotinic acid — the tongue is swollen and the red color of raw beef. Deficiency produces inflammation of the gums, inflammation of the mouth and an inflamed tongue.

Pyridoxine — deficiency characterized by cracking of the lips and corners of the mouth; inflammation of the tongue. Symptoms may be due to generalized B complex deficiency rather than specifically pyridoxine.

Vitamin $B_{12}$ — the smooth, sore tongue associated with deficiency is almost diagnostic since it is usually a feature of pernicious anemia.

Vitamin C — in a severe deficiency there are bleeding gums, inflamed gums and a loosening of the teeth. Small localized hemorrhages appear in the mouth.

Biotin — in infants suffering from the specific dermatitis associated with deficiency there is also rawness of the surface of the mouth.

*The gastro-intestinal tract* — can be affected by vitamin B complex deficiency at any level.

Thiamine — deficiency characterized by diarrhea, accompanied by abdominal distention and stomach pains.

Nicotinic acid — deficiency invariably gives rise to diarrhea.

Pantothenic acid — paralysis of parts of the intestinal tract including post-operative paralytic ileus may be associated with deficiency. Symptoms are abdominal distress and distension, sometimes with the inability to pass motions.

*The eye* — deficiencies can affect both sight and eye tissues.

Vitamin A — specific symptom of deficiency is night blindness characterized by poor adaptation of the eye to low-intensity light conditions. Eye tissue is also thickened and dry, particularly that of the cornea (white of the eye) and conjunctiva (mucous membranes).

Riboflavin — white of the eye (cornea) develops prominent redness due to blood vessels; conjunctivitis (inflammation of the mucous membranes) is common in the lower lid; feeling of grittiness in the eye; constant watering and failing vision are symptoms of deficiency.

Thiamine — most common symptom of deficiency in eye is dimness of vision not associated with a specific lesion of the eye. Other ocular signs include involuntary rhythmic movement of the eyeballs, known as nystagmus; eye muscle fatigue; paralysis of the eye with loss of visual activity (acuteness or clearness).

Nicotinic acid — symptoms are very similar to those associated with thiamine deficiency suggesting they are multivitamin-deficient in origin.

Vitamin C — hemorrhages inside the eye often appear before those on the skin.

Vitamin K — when lacking in the newborn, often induces hemorrhages in the retina.

*The central nervous system* — deficiency of most of the B vitamins causes symptoms associated with the nerves.

Thiamine — gross deficiency causes mental confusion leading to coma. Milder deficiency gives rise to nystagmus (involuntary rhythmic movement of the eyeballs) and sometimes mental confusion. Other mental symptoms include narration of fictitious experiences (confabulation) and polyneuritis (nerve inflammation). Nervous consequences include foot and wrist drop when motor nerves are involved.

Pyridoxine — in infants deficiency has been found to produce convulsions due to inadequate level of GABA (gamma aminobutyric acid) in brain. In adults most usual symptom is generalized inflammation of the nerves (peripheral neuritis) characterized by tingling, numbness, burning pain and loss of vibratory sensation.

Nicotinic acid — early signs are peripheral neuritis (see above) and encephalopathy (brain disease or inflammation). Later symptoms are due to progressive dementia characterized by apprehension, confusion, derangement and maniacal outbursts.

Vitamin $B_{12}$ — symptoms of deficiency are pins and needles in feet and hands, weakness in the limbs, leg stiffness, unsteadiness, lethargy and fatigue. Delirium and confusion are seen in advanced cases. Tactile (touch) sensation is impaired and reflexes are depressed.

Folic acid — only mental deficiency symptom is psychosis characterized by mental derangement in which the patient is confused and lacks ability to describe events and is unaware of symptoms.

*The blood* — various vitamins when deficient give rise to anemias of different types. Symptoms of all anemias are similar and include paleness, tiredness, lethargy, breathlessness, weakness, vertigo, headache, tinnitus (constant noises in the head), spots before the eyes, drowsiness, irritability, amenorrhea, loss of libido and sometimes low-grade fever. Occasionally gastro-intestinal complaints and even heart failure may develop.

Particular type of anemia requires blood and sometimes bone-marrow examination for correct diagnosis and must be left to medical practitioner.

Hypochromic anemia — characterized by red blood cells depleted of hemoglobin. May be caused by deficiency of pyridoxine or riboflavin. Sometimes complicated by small red blood cells also when it is known as microcytic hypochromic anemia.

Megaloblastic anemia — characterized by excessive numbers of immature red cells in the blood that cannot function as oxygen-carriers. May be caused by deficiency of folic acid or vitamin $B_{12}$.

Iron-deficiency anemia — characterized by inability to produce hemoglobin because of lack of iron. If vitamin C is deficient, iron cannot be absorbed or incorporated into hemoglobin. Vitamin C deficiency also causes hemorrhage so this too may contribute to the anemia.

Hemolytic anemia — characterized by unstable red blood cells that burst readily and have short life. May be caused by vitamin E deficiency in infants and adults.

The heart and blood vessels — thiamine deficiency in later stages causes severely weakened heart muscle leading to circulatory failure. The heart is grossly enlarged. Vitamin $B_6$ deficiency may give rise to massive deposition of fats in the heart and blood vessels, known as atherosclerosis.

*The bones* — changes in the bones due to vitamin deficiency can usually be detected by X-ray diagnosis and clinical diagnosis only. Some changes, such as those produced by deficiency in vitamin A, riboflavin, pyridoxine and pantothenic acid, have been noted only in animals.

Vitamin C — deficiency produces irregular calcification but this is obvious only from X-ray examinations.

Vitamin D — deficiency in infants causes rickets, the most obvious signs of which are: restlessness and inability to sleep; retarded ability to sit, crawl or walk; retarded closure and hardening of the skull bones due to lack of mineralization. The long bones fail to ossify and are unable to stand the weight of the child so that they bend, leading to bow-legs and knock-knees. Pigeon-breast deformity is sometimes obvious. These changes are detected earlier in X-ray examination.

Deficiency of vitamin D in adults leads to ostomalacia, different to rickets because in the adult disease the bones are pre-formed. Demineralization occurs rather than a failure to mineralize the bones. Bones affected are spine, pelvis and lower extremities. As bones soften, the legs may become bowed, the vertebrae shortens (reducing the height) and the pelvic bones flatten.

*The reproductive system* — vitamin deficiencies in most animal species induce changes in the reproductive organs and process. In the females fetal abnormalities sometimes resulting in abortion are symptoms of deficiency. No exact parallel in human beings but there are scattered reports that vitamin $B_{12}$ or vitamin E deficiency can produce sterility in males and miscarriage in females, reversible by appropriate vitamin therapy.

---

**deficiency tests,** deficiencies in vitamins are usually determined from blood tests but these are normally taken only in conjunction with clinical signs before a medical diagnosis of deficiency is accepted. Hair analysis cannot indicate the vitamin status of an individual but it does give a clue to possible mineral deficiencies. Tests for vitamin deficiency are as follows:

*Vitamin A* — the level of this and of carotene can be determined in the blood but neither measurement is a good indication of body status of these vitamins, since there is considerable storage of each in the body. Normal vitamin A concentration is between 15 and 60µg per 100ml blood serum; that of carotene is between 8 and 40µg per 100ml blood serum.

*Vitamin D* — the best diagnostic procedure to determine vitamin D deficiency is to estimate 25-hydroxycholecalciferol in the blood but it is a specialized assay. Radiographic examination is a good way to detect rickets and osteomalacia in individuals, particularly X-ray pictures of the ends of the long bones. A third test is to measure the blood concentration of the enzyme alkaline phosphatase — high levels may indicate rickets even before the X-ray changes prove it but this test is not specific.

*Vitamin E* — there are three tests that can indicate a possible vitamin E deficiency; first, the measurement of blood serum tocopherol levels is simple and a reliable index of the circulating vitamin. Normal values lie between 1.0 and 3.0mg per 100ml blood serum.

The second test involves measuring the creatine content of the patients' urines. Usually this is absent from urine but when vitamin E is deficient, creatine appears in the urine. Creatine, usually excreted as creatinine, comes from the muscles and excess amount in the urine is indicative of muscle breakdown which is a function of vitamin E deficiency.

The third test involves measuring the fragility of the red blood cells in the presence of hydrogen peroxide. Normal red blood cells are resistant to hydrogen peroxide but when they are vitamin E-deficient they readily burst in the presence of the peroxide. Such tests are carried out on isolated blood.

*Vitamin K* — this is impossible to measure directly in the blood but an indication of vitamin K status comes from assay of the levels of the clotting factors of the blood. The usual test is to measure prothrombin time which gives a reasonable estimation of the vitamin K present. This test is also used to monitor the effect of the vitamin K antagonists like warfarin on the clotting of the blood when the drugs are being taken regularly.

*Vitamin C* — possible deficiency can be indicated by a combination of blood plasma levels and the extent of urinary excretion of the vitamin. White blood cell levels of vitamin C are a better indication of blood levels than those of plasma but the technique is time-consuming and is used more in research than as a standard technique. Normal blood levels of vitamin C are from 0.4 to 1.5mg per 100ml but white blood cells contain from 25 to 38mg per 100ml. A level of below 7mg per 100ml white blood cells indicates a high risk of scurvy.

Normally only 13 to 15mg of vitamin C is excreted daily in the urine; less than this indicates a possible deficiency. Confirmation usually comes from a saturation test. Multiple small doses of the vitamin are given over a period of time. Four to six hours after these, the urine level of the vitamin is measured. If the individual is suffering from vitamin C deficiency urine levels will not rise because the body saturates its tissues before excreting any. Hence the appearance of greater-than-normal amounts of the vitamin in the urine suggests the body is saturated and hence there is no deficiency. If none is excreted, vitamin C intakes are increased until the vitamin appears in the urine. An individual can easily determine if he or she needs vitamin C by carrying out the above test on himself. A dose of 300mg every 4 to 6 hours is taken in water. Vitamin C is assessed in the urine by adding a dye to a sample of the urine. If the dye is decolorized vitamin C is present. A suitable dye is 2, 4-dinitrophenyl hydrazine, available impregnated into paper dipsticks. A mass screening test involves introducing a harmless blue dye, 2, 6-dichlorophenolindophenol, onto the tongue or just beneath the surface of the gum. The time taken for the dye to decolorize reflects the vitamin C status of the body — the longer the time the more chance of deficiency of the vitamin. The test is simply a preliminary one and must be confirmed by other means before a diagnosis can be made of true vitamin C deficiency.

*Thiamine* — can be measured directly in the blood and urine or indirectly by assaying an enzyme dependent on the vitamin for activity. Blood plasma levels are very low under normal conditions at concentration between 0.5

and 1.3µg per 100ml. Measurement of the vitamin excreted in a 24-hour urine sample is a reliable indication of thiamine deficiency. It can be improved in sensitivity by measuring urinary excretion after taking an oral dose of the vitamin. If this stays low, there is a good chance that the individual is lacking thiamine.

*Riboflavin* — the usual criteria for determining if a patient is deficient in riboflavin are the medical history, clinical examination and response to therapy with the vitamin. Red blood cell determinations are not easy because the normal level is very low, between 20 and 28µg per 100ml. For this reason an enzyme, glutathione reluctase, that requires riboflavin, is usually assayed to indicate riboflavin levels.

*Pyridoxine* — the amount of pyridoxal phosphate present in the blood before and after an oral dose of the vitamin can be indicative of deficiency of the vitamin. Normal levels are at least 5µg per 100ml. A second test involves measuring xanthurenic acid in the urine. Normally this is less than 25mg per day but if an oral dose of the amino acid tryptophane is given to an individual who is deficient in pyridoxine, xanthurenic acid is excreted at levels greater than 50mg per day. Pyridoxine is necessary to convert xanthurenic acid further in body metabolism, so in the absence of the vitamin this compound builds up and is readily excreted.

*Nicotinic acid* — blood measurements are not reliable because no test is sufficiently sensitive or specific. Assay is usually carried out by measuring the ratio of methyl nicotinic derivatives to creatinine in the urine.

*Vitamin $B_{12}$* — blood levels can be measured directly using the fact that some bacteria need the vitamin for normal growth. The extent of growth of the micro-organism indicates the amount of vitamin $B_{12}$ present in a sample of blood. Normal blood levels are 0.015 to 0.03µg per 100ml blood plasma. Levels below 0.01µg per 100ml are indicative of vitamin $B_{12}$ deficiency.

The more usual test for deficiency involves radio-activity labelled $B_{12}$ to measure its absorption. This is described under Schilling Test.

*Folic acid* — a diagnosis of deficiency is usually assessed on the basis of a macrocytic anemia (in the absence of $B_{12}$ deficiency), a megaloblastic bone marrow and leucopenia (low white blood cell count). Blood serum levels can be measured but are difficult and time-consuming on a routine basis. Normal values are 0.5 to 2.0µg per 100ml in serum; 16 to 64µg per 100ml red blood cells. When the amino acid histidine is given orally, the quantity of formimino-glutamic acid (FIGLU) in the urine is increased dramatically in folic acid deficiency. This test is usually carried out in conjunction with the other tests mentioned above.

*Pantothenic acid* — measurement of the pantothenic acid level in the blood alone is usually indicative of deficiency of this vitamin. Confirmation usually comes from measuring coenzyme A activity which contains and is dependent on pantothenic acid levels.

---

**dehydroretinol,**   $A_2$ vitamin.

---

**delta tocopherol,**   *see* E vitamin.

---

**deodorant,**   vitamin E included as antioxidant to retard degradation of oxygen-containing components of sweat.

---

**deoxyribonucleic acids,**   DNA. Nucleic acids, constituents of all cells, essential for synthesis of protein and transmission of hereditary characteristics to offspring. The basis of life's processes, lack of DNA production has profound effects on health, first sign of which is megalogblastic anemia, and process of ageing.

   Vitamins essential for DNA synthesis are A, folic acid, $B_6$, $B_{12}$, E and choline. Abnormal DNA metabolism may be related to cancer.

---

**depression,**   mild variety can be related to vitamin $B_6$ deficiency induced by drugs, contraceptive pill or premenstrual tension (PMT). Treated with 25 to 50mg $B_6$ daily or 50 to 100mg from day 10 of one menstrual cycle to day 3 of the next when due to PMT or contraceptive pill. When associated with drugs need at least 25mg $B_6$ daily.

---

**dermatitis,**   inflammation of the skin characterized by redness, oozing, crusting, scaling and sometimes blisters. May be related to lack of vitamin B complex, vitamin A or vitamin F. Treated with whole B complex at high potency; vitamin A, both oral and topical; PUFA orally, especially safflower oil or oil of evening primrose.

---

**desiccated liver,**   concentrated beef liver powder which has been dried in vacuum at a low temperature to conserve original nutrient value of the liver.

Vitamins present (in mg per 100g) are: vitamin A (20mg); thiamine (1.0); riboflavin (9.57); pyridoxine (2.31); nicotinic acid (44.9); pantothenic acid (24.1); folic acid (1.09); vitamin $B_{12}$ (0.363); biotin (0.109); vitamin C (75.9); vitamin E (1.39); carotene (5.08).

---

**diabetes mellitus,** associated with high blood sugar level that persists long after meals because of lack of hormone insulin. Long-term consequences are arteriosclerosis, heart disease, gangrene, blindness that may be related to specific vitamin deficiencies. Increased requirements for vitamins $B_6$ (25mg), C (500mg), E (400IU), A (7500IU) (because diabetics cannot produce it from carotenes), daily.

---

**diarrhea,** specifically associated with severe deficiency of nicotinamide but may respond to supplementation with whole vitamin B complex.

---

**Dickerson, Professor J. W. T.,** British biochemist. Professor of Human Nutrition, University of Surrey, Guildford, UK, leading researcher in vitamin C and cancer and in the effect of medicinal drugs on nutritional status.

---

**dicoumarol,** anti-coagulant drug which acts by inhibiting action of vitamin K.

---

**digestive tract,** gastro-intestinal tract. Stomach and intestines where digestion of food and absorption of nutrients takes place.

Nicotinamide (at doses up to 3000mg daily) has been used to treat malabsorption diseases of the intestine such as sprue. Folic acid deficiency can destroy lining cells of the small intestine and impair absorption process. Lack of pantothenic acid can cause abdominal distension. Supplementary vitamin can reduce post-operative distension and nausea including effects of paralytic ileus. Thiamine promotes good digestion and better functioning of the digestive tract. Improves muscles of the tract and can cure stubborn cases of constipation.

Vitamin C, when taken with aspirin, can prevent gastric bleeding induced by the drug. Gastric ulcers can be prevented by high doses of vitamin E (up to 600IU daily). Better results with vitamin A which at high doses (150000IU daily for four weeks) has been used to treat gastric ulcers. Indications that prevention of stomach cancer may benefit from vitamin A supplementation.

---

**disease resistance,** depends on efficiency of development of immune response which requires adequate vitamin A, folic acid, vitamin B$_{12}$, vitamin C, pantothenic acid and choline.

---

**Donath, W. F.,** *see* Jansen, B. C. P.

---

**dried apricots,** *in the raw state,* provide higher quantities of the vitamins (except vitamin C and thiamine) compared with fresh fruit. Carotene content is 3.6mg per 100g (range 2.4-4.4mg) but negligible vitamin E. B vitamins present (in mg per 100g) are: thiamine 0.01; riboflavin 0.20; nicotinic acid 3.8; pyridoxine 0.17; pantothenic acid 0.70. Folic acid level is 14μg per 100g; biotin is absent. Vitamin C is destroyed by drying the fruit so only traces are left.

*When stewed,* with or without sugar, all vitamin levels are reduced because of uptake of water. Carotene content is 1.3mg per 100g but no vitamin E present. B vitamins present are (in mg per 100g): thiamine 0.01; riboflavin 0.06; nicotinic acid 1.4; pyridoxine 0.05; pantothenic acid 0.23. Folic acid drastically reduced to 2μg per 100g.

*When canned,* most vitamin levels are reduced further compared with those in stewed fruit. Carotene content is 1.0mg per 100g. B vitamins present are (in mg per 100g): thiamine 0.02; riboflavin 0.01; nicotinic acid 0.4; pyridoxine 0.05; pantothenic acid 0.10. Folic acid level is 5μg per 100g.

---

**dried currants,** provide 30μg carotene per 100g. Vitamin E cannot be detected. B vitamins present are (in mg per 100g): thiamine 0.03; riboflavin 0.08; nicotinic acid 0.6; pyridoxine 0.30; pantothenic acid 0.10. Folic acid can be detected in dried fruit at level of 11μg per 100g. Vitamin C destroyed completely during drying process.

---

**dried figs,** more concentrated source of B vitamins than fresh figs, but stewing reduces the potency, with and without sugar addition. Carotene levels for raw figs, stewed without sugar and stewed with sugar respectively are (in µg per 100g) 50, 30, 30. Vitamin E is absent. B vitamins present (in mg per 100g), for the raw fruit, stewed without sugar and stewed with sugar respectively, are: thiamine 0.10, 0.05, 0.05; riboflavin 0.08, 0.04, 0.04; nicotinic acid 2.2, 1.2, 1.2; pyridoxine 0.18, 0.08, 0.07; pantothenic acid 0.44, 0.22, 0.21. Folic acid levels (in µg per 100g) are respectively 9, 2 and 2. Biotin is absent. No vitamin C present.

---

**dried peaches,**   higher potency of all vitamins, except vitamin C, compared with fresh fruit. Some losses of vitamins on stewing, with and without sugar. Carotene content is high at 2.0mg per 100g; when stewed without sugar and with sugar, level is reduced to 740 and 710µg per 100g respectively. Vitamin E has not been detected. B vitamins present are (in mg per 100g), for raw, edible portion, stewed without sugar and stewed with sugar respectively: thiamine, traces only; riboflavin 0.19, 0.06, 0.06; nicotinic acid 5.6, 2.1, 2.0; pyridoxine 0.10, 0.03, 0.03; pantothenic acid 0.30, 0.10, 0.10. Folic acid levels are respectively 14, 2 and 2µg per 100g. Biotin has not been detected. Traces only of vitamin C in dried peaches.

---

**dried peas,**   in the raw state represent good sources of B vitamins and carotene that are reduced on boiling, due to losses and to uptake of water. Levels of carotene (in µg per 100g) are, in the raw and boiled state respectively, 250 and 80. Traces only of vitamin E. Levels of B vitamins are (in mg per 100g), in the raw and boiled state respectively: thiamine 0.60, 0.11; riboflavin 0.30, 0.07; nicotinic acid 6.5, 2.1; pyridoxine 0.13, undetected; pantothenic acid 2.0, undetected. Folic acid present to the extent of 33µg per 100g in dried state but not detected in boiled peas. Traces only of vitamin C.

---

**dried potatoes,**   retain good levels of vitamins but these are reduced when prepared for eating because of addition of water. B vitamins present (in mg per 100g), in dried and made-up mash respectively are: thiamine 0.04, 0.01; riboflavin 0.14, 0.03; nicotinic acid 7.8, 1.7; pyridoxine 0.82, 0.18; pantothenic acid 0.91, 0.20. Folic acid levels are respectively 25 and 4µg per 100g respectively. Biotin levels are 0.5 and 0.1µg per 100g respectively. Contribute 12 and 3mg vitamin C per 100g respectively. However when fortified with the vitamin, these levels may increase ten-fold.

---

**drinking chocolate,** useful source of some vitamins. Figures are for the dry form. Vitamin E content is 0.9mg per 100g. B vitamins present are (in mg per 100g): thiamine 0.06; riboflavin 0.04; nicotinic acid 1.1; pyridoxine 0.02. Folic acid level is 10$\mu$g per 100g. Devoid of vitamin C.

---

**dripping,** beef fat. Contains no vitamin A, carotene or vitamin C. Traces only of all the B vitamins.

---

**drugs,** may increase requirements for certain vitamins; may cause malabsorption of vitamins; may interfere with utilization and activation of vitamins. See individual drugs.

---

**dry skin,** increase intake of vitamin A (7500IU daily) and PUFA (safflower oil, wheatgerm oil or oil of evening primrose up to 3g daily) and lecithin (up to 6 capsules daily). Treat affected area with vitamin E cream.

---

# E

---

**E,** tocopherol from "tokos" birth and "phero" to bear. Fat-soluble vitamin. Known also as d-alpha tocopherol (natural); dl-alpha tocopherol (synthetic); d-beta tocopherol, d-gamma tocopherol, d-delta tocopherol (all natural); anti-sterility vitamin; fertility vitamin. Isolated from wheatgerm oil by Drs. H. M. Evans and K. S. Bishop in 1936 at University of California. Present in supplements as d-alpha tocopheryl acetate, d-alpha tocopheryl succinate (both natural); dl-alpha tocopheryl acetate, dl-alpha tocopheryl succinate (both synthetic). Also may be present as d-alpha tocopherol (natural) and dl-alpha tocopherol (synthetic). Available as water-solubilized vitamin. Foods contain mixture of all four tocopherols.

*Richest food sources* (in mg per 100g) are (total tocopherols:d-alpha tocopherol) wheat germ oil (190:139); soybean oil (87.1:9.1); tung-oil (81.0:24.3); corn oil (66.1:10.1); cottonseed oil (63.5:31.8); safflower oil (49.2:23.8); rice bran oil (44.4:26.2); sunflower oil (27.1:24.2); peanut oil

(21.5:7.7); cod liver oil (20.0:20.0); roasted peanuts (11.7:7.7); potato chips (11.4:6.4); peanut butter (7.7:6.0); fried onion rings (6.4:0.7); shrimps (6.6:0.6); linseed oil (6.1:0); olive oil (4.6:4.6); egg-yolk (4.6:1.6); granola (3.2:1.7); brown rice (2.4:1.2); turnip greens (2.24:2.19); salmon steak (1.81:1.35); fresh peas (1.73:0.55); green beans (1.68:0.47); liver (1.62:0.63); french fries (1.59:0.42); tomatoes (1.40:1.20); meats (0.63:0.37); celery (0.57:0.38); apples (0.51:0.31); bananas (0.42:0.22); strawberries (0.4:0.21); oranges (0.23:0.22); onion (0.34:0.22); carrots (0.50:0.50); lettuce (1.20:0.50); potatoes (0.09:0.05).

*Destroyed substantially by* commercial cooking and processing of foods including deep freezing. Home cooking losses much less except for deep-frying. Solvent extraction of grain and seed oils destroys the vitamin but this is preserved by cold-pressing of oils. Destroyed by *ferric* iron but not by *ferrous* iron.

*Functions* essentially as antioxidant and hence has protective action but in addition it reduces the oxygen requirements of muscles and organs; acts as an anti-blood-clotting agent; dissolves blood clots; opens up new channels of blood supply; causes smaller blood vessels to dilate; strengthens blood capillary walls; helps to regenerate new skin; helps in process of normal clotting of blood; improves the action of insulin in diabetes; acts as a diuretic; increases power and activity of muscles; neutralizes the effect of harmful free radicals; acts as antipollutant; protects polyunsaturated fatty acids; protects sulphur-containing amino acids; protects vitamin A; prevents thrombosis; prevents atherosclerosis; prevents thrombophlebitis; increases proportion of HDL-cholesterol; acts in conjunction with selenium; mutually protects vitamin C; increases ability of white blood cells to resist infection.

*Deficiency in man* does not give rise to specific disease apart from anemia in new-born babies. Develops from: inefficient absorption of fats due to intestinal disease; pancreatic disease; gastric or intestinal surgery; alcoholism; cirrhosis of the liver; obstructive jaundice; cystic fibrosis; tropical sprue; celiac disease; excessive intake of polyunsaturated fats, excessive oxygen as in oxygen tents; excessive intake of mineral oils, e.g. liquid paraffin.

*Symptoms of deficiency* in premature infants and children are irritability, edema (retention of water) and hemolytic anemia. In adults there is lack of vitality, lethargy, apathy, inability to concentrate, irritability, disinterest in physical activity, decreased sexual performance, muscle weakness. Deposition of brown fat in body organs.

*Deficiency in animals* causes muscular dystrophy in all species; degeneration of the testes in rats, rabbits, dogs and fowl; fetal resorption in the rat; nerve degeneration in rats, fowl, cattle and monkeys; heart and blood circulation defects in all species; eczema, urticaria and itching in poultry; respiratory infections in poultry; exudative diathesis in poultry; increased tendency of blood cells to burst; excessive urinary excretion of creatine in all species; yellow fat disease in cat, pig and poultry.

Recommended dietary intakes in the USA are 10IU for children under 4 years and 30IU for anyone over 4 years, including pregnant and lactating women. Intakes have not been set by the UK and WHO.

*Increased intakes* required in: any malabsorption disease; in liver disease; following surgery of the digestive tract; in obstructive jaundice; in cystic fibrosis; in tropical sprue; in celiac disease; in increased intake of polyunsaturated fats and oils; during long-term treatment with liquid paraffin; during excessive oxygen inhalation; in diabetes; during infectious disease. There is no limit in the USA or UK on supplementary doses of the vitamin.

*Toxicity symptoms* are muscle weakness and proneness to fatigue. There may be transient increase in blood-pressure with palpitations of the heart. No blood-pressure increase in those on heart drugs. Oily nature of vitamin may cause nausea and mild diarrhea. Toxicity symptoms very rare at daily doses up to 600IU. Only occasional reports at daily intakes between 600IU and 1000IU. Doses greater than 1000IU daily should be taken under medical supervision.

*Therapy* has been found to be beneficial in: intermittent claudication; cerebral thrombosis; coronary thrombosis; atherosclerosis; arteriosclerosis; varicose veins; thrombophlebitis; menstrual problems; sterility; intractable ulcers of the skin; gangrene induced by diabetes; treatment of sunburn; treatment of scalding; nerve, joint and muscular complaints; anemia of the new-born; thalassemia minor and major; sickle-cell anemia; prevention of blindness in premature babies; cystic breast disease; breast cancer.

---

**eczema,** acute or chronic non-contagious itching, inflammatory disease of the skin. Can be due to essential fatty acids (EFA) deficiency, but more specifically that of gamma linolenic acid (GLA).

*Infantile* eczema may be due to lack of GLA in cow's milk. Treat with oral oil of evening primrose (1500 to 3000mg daily).

*Atopic* eczema due to allergic reaction. Shown to respond to oral oil of evening primrose (up to 3000mg daily).

Other vitamin treatment includes vitamin A (7500IU), vitamin C (up to 1000mg) and high potency vitamin B complex including inositol (500mg daily).

---

**edema,** retention of excessive water in the body. Not a disease in its own right but a symptom of some other complaint. Has been claimed that high potencies of certain vitamins have a diuretic effect in removing excess water: vitamin C at levels of one gram or more. May be effective for mild edema, e.g. in premenstrual syndrome, but most edema requires stronger acting drugs (medicinal or herbal).

**eggplant,** virtually devoid of fat-soluble vitamins. B vitamins present (in mg per 100g) include: thiamine 0.05; riboflavin 0.03; nicotinic acid 0.9; pyridoxine 0.08; pantothenic acid 0.22. Folic acid present at concentrations of $20\mu g$ per 100g.

**eggs,** moderate source of all vitamins except vitamin C. *Whole, raw* provide (in mg per 100g): vitamin A 0.14; carotene, trace, thiamine 0.09; riboflavin 0.47; nicotinic acid 3.68; pyridoxine 0.11; folic acid 0.025; pantothenic acid 1.8; biotin 0.025; vitamin $B_{12}$ 0.0017; vitamin E 1.6. *Raw egg-white* is completely devoid of all fat-soluble vitamins.

The percentage losses of vitamins in cooked eggs are whon in Table 7.

**Table 7: Percentage losses of vitamins in cooking eegs**

|  | Thiamine | Riboflavin | Pyridoxine | Folic acid | Pantothenic acid |
|---|---|---|---|---|---|
| Boiled | 10 | 5 | 10 | 10 | 10 |
| Fried | 20 | 10 | 20 | 30 | 20 |
| Poached | 20 | 20 | 20 | 35 | 20 |
| Omelette | 5 | 20 | 15 | 30 | 15 |
| Scrambled | 5 | 20 | 15 | 30 | 15 |

**elderly,** largest single group of population prone to mild deficiency of vitamins, particularly B complex C and K. Reasons include aversion to salads and meat because of poor dentition; reluctance for physical or emotional reasons to shop frequently for a variety of foods; loss of marital partner with less care in preparing food because of apathy; undue reliance on refined carbohydrates and simple beverages as staple diet; dependence on restaurant or institutional cooking; inefficient absorption of food micronutrients.

Most elderly persons will benefit from daily multivitamin supplement with extra vitamin C (250-500mg) plus choline as phosphatidyl choline (3-6 capsules daily) or lecithin (5-15g) daily to improve mental activity.

---

**Elvehjem, Conrad,** Dutch doctor who, at the University of Wisconsin, USA, first identified the pellagra-preventing factor as nicotinic acid in 1937.

---

**embolism,** obstruction or occlusion of a blood vessel, especially an artery, by a transported clot. Treatment, *see* blood clot.

---

**endive,** a kind of chicory. Good source of carotene, contributing 2mg per 100g on average, but supplies only traces of vitamin E. Levels of B vitamins present (in mg per 100g) are: thiamine 0.05; riboflavin 0.05; nicotinic acod 0.6. Excellent source of folic acid at 330μg per 100g. Contributes 12mg vitamin C per 100g endive.

---

**endurance,** increased by vitamin E. Optimum daily intake of 100-150IU for training period of 1.5-2.0 hours; 250-300IU for training period of 3-4 hours.

In racehorses, daily intakes of 5000-10000IU vitamin E have increased performance and calmed nervous animals.

---

**enteritis,** regional. *See* Crohn's disease.

---

**epilepsy,** convulsive seizures. Large amounts of folic acod may neutralize action of anti-convulsive drugs, particularly phenytoin.

---

**etretinate,** vitamin A-related, synthetic derivative of retinoic acid used in treating psoriasis and other skin disorders by oral route.

Side-effects include dryness of mucous membranes and hair loss. Teratogenic (causing abnormal fetus), so pregnancy must be avoided during use. Strict medical use only.

---

**Evans, H. M.,** American scientist who with K. S. Bishop discovered vitamin E in 1923 at the University of California, finally isolating it from wheat germ oil in 1936. Coined the name tocopherol.

---

**extrinsic factor,** *see* $B_{12}$ vitamin.

---

**eyes,** sight process depends upon adequate vitamin A (2500IU daily). Bloodshot eyes prevented by vitamin $B_2$ (10mg daily). Heavy smoking causes tobacco amblyopia (reduced vision) due to inactivation of vitamin $B_{12}$.

# F

---

**farnoquinone,** $K_2$ vitamin.

---

**fatigue,** early sign of deficiency of pantothenic acid; of thiamine; of vitamin C; of vitamin E. May be associated with generalized mild deficiency of vitamins. Treat with multivitamin preparation. If no improvement after one month seek medical advice.

---

**fats,** complexes of fatty acids, both polyunsaturated (vitamin F) and saturated, and glycerine. Hard fats usually contain mainly saturated and mono-unsaturated fatty acids (e.g. fats of animal origin); oils usually contain mainly polyunsaturated with some mono-unsaturated fatty acids (e.g. vegetable oils). Hard margarines are mainly saturated and monosaturated fatty acids; soft margarines contain more polyunsaturated fatty acids.

All fats and oils of whatever origin provide 9 k calories per gram. Dietary fats in Western world provide about 40 per cent of total calorie intake. Most authorities now recommend reduction to between 25 and 35 per cent of total calorie intake. Some suggest replacement of saturated fats in diet to polyunsaturated variety by switching from animal fats to vegetable oils. High polyunsaturated fat intake requires increased vitamin E concomitantly.

High blood fats can be reduced with vitamin E (400IU) and vitamin C (500mg) and soy lecithin granules (15g) daily. Lecithin provides 120 kilocalories in 15g that must be counted against fat intake. High blood fats associated with high fat intake regarded as increasing chances of developing cancer, gout, coronary thrombosis, stroke and complications of diabetes.

---

**fatty acids,** metabolism dependent on vitamin $B_2$; vitamin C (via carnitine in muscle cells). *See* fats and polyunsaturated fatty acids (vitamin F).

---

**fertility,** measured in men by number and mobility of spermatozoa in semen. No definite association in men between infertility and vitamin deficiency but some evidence that vitamins A, $B_{12}$ and E needed for normal sperm production. These vitamins definitely required by many species of animals for reproduction. No strong evidence that vitamin E can help infertile human females but 200IU daily has prevented miscarriage in those prone to it. Vitamin $B_{12}$ can also help some women unable to conceive.

---

**figs,** in the raw, green state are good source of carotene, with some B vitamins and a little vitamin C. Carotene content is 500µg per 100g but vitamin E is absent. B vitamins present (in mg per 100g) are: thiamine 0.06; riboflavin 0.05; nicotinic acid 0.6; pyridoxine 0.11; pantothenic acid 0.30. Folic acid and biotin were not detectable. *See also* dried figs.

---

**fish,** *white variety* includes cod, haddock, Atlantic halibut, lemon sole, plaice, saithe and whiting. All contain only traces of vitamin A, D and carotene but Pacific halibut has 120µg vitamin A and 1µg vitamin D per 100g. Vitamin E potencies vary from 0.36 to 1.0mg per 100g.

All are moderate sources of the B vitamins and concentrations (in mg per 100g) are in the range: thiamine 0.06-0.30; riboflavin 0.05-0.22; nicotinic acid 2.4-9.6; pyridoxine 0.17-0.62; pantothenic acid 0.13-0.80. All contain vitamin $B_{12}$ at levels between 1 and 5µg per 100g plus traces of folic acid (3-16μg per 100g) and biotin (2-5μg per 100g).

Vitamin C content of all white fish is negligible. Plaice tends to contain the higher levels of those quoted.

*Fatty variety* includes eel, herring, bloater, kipper, mackerel, pilchard, salmon, sardines, sprats, trout, tuna and whitebait. Eel is rich source of vitamin A at 1.9mg per 100g, but herring, bloater, kipper and mackerel supply less (26-52μg per 100g) while others supply only traces. Eel body oil contains 120μg vitamin D per 100g. Herring, bloater, kipper and mackerel are good sources of vitamin D, supplying between 13.5 and 25.0μg per 100g. Other fatty fish contain only traces of vitamin D.

All fatty fish are poor sources of thiamine with the exception of salmon, which contains up to 0.20mg per 100g (canned has only 0.04μg). Other B vitamins are present in moderate concentrations which are (in mg per 100g): riboflavin 0.1-0.4; nicotinic acid 2.3-13.1; pyridoxine 0.24-0.84; pantothenic acid 0.15-0.84. Good levels of vitamin $B_{12}$ from 5 to 28μg per 100g; traces of folic acid (up to 15μg) and biotin (up to 10μg).

Canned tuna in oil supplies 9.2mg vitamin E per 100g and salmon up to 1.5mg but others are poor sources with less than 0.3mg per 100g fish. Traces only of vitamin C in all fatty fish.

*Losses of vitamins* during the cooking of fish are shown in Table 8 as percentages.

**Table 8: Percentage losses of vitamins during the cooking of fish.**

|  | *Poaching* | *Baking* | *Frying/broiling* |
|---|---|---|---|
| Thiamine | 10 | 30 | 20 |
| Riboflavin | 0 | 20 | 20 |
| Nicotinic acid | 10 | 20 | 20 |
| Pyridoxine | 0 | 10 | 20 |
| Pantothenic acid | 20 | 20 | 20 |
| Folic acid | 50 | 20 | 0 |
| Vitamin $B_{12}$ | 0 | 10 | 0 |
| Biotin | 10 | 10 | 10 |
| Vitamin C | 5 | 5 | 20 |
| Vitamin E | 0 | 0 | 0 |

**fish sticks,** poor sources of all the vitamins. Traces only of vitamin A, carotene, D and E. B vitamins present only to the extent (in mg per 100g) of: thiamine 0.08; riboflavin 0.06; nicotinic acid 3.6; pyridoxine 0.21.

Vitamin $B_{12}$ level is $1\mu g$ per 100g; folic acid $15\mu g$. Vitamin C is absent.

---

**fish oils,**　fish body oils as well as fish liver oils are rich sources of PUFA but also two especially that are not found in vegetable seed oils. These are EPA (eicosapentaenoic acid) and DHA (docosahexaenoic acid). Both are essential fatty acids (part of vitamin F complex) that function as precursors of the hormones known as prostaglandins. These prostaglandins are believed to inhibit formation of blood clots in the circulatory system; reduce blood fat levels; increase HDL-cholesterol levels and reduce risk of heart disease and stroke. They effectively thin the blood. Daily intake of ½-1 lb of oily fish (such as mackerel or herring) supplies sufficient EPA and DHA for protective effect. Cod-liver oil will supply them but too risky because of vitamins A and D content.

Supplements now available that provide EPA (180mg) and DHA (120mg) per capsule that doubles usual daily intake. Preventative therapy requires up to 3 capsules daily (900mg total EPA and DHA). For those with angina or who have suffered heart attacks or stroke, five daily is sufficient (1500mg total EPA and DHA) to help prevent further attacks.

---

**folacin,**　*see* folic acid.

---

**folates,**　group of folic-acid-related compounds that occurs in foods only some of which show vitamin activity.

---

**folic acid,**　water-soluble vitamin, member of the vitamin B complex. Also known as vitamin Bc; vitamin M; pteroyl glutamic acid, PGA; liver lactobacillus casei factor; folacin. Anti-anemia vitamin. Present in supplements as folic acid and calcium folinate. Yellow-orange crystalline powder.

Anti-anemia factor for monkeys found in yeast and liver in 1935 designated vitamin M. In 1939 anti-anemia factor for chicks isolated from liver called vitamin Bc. In 1940 growth factor for lactobacillus casei and growth factor for streptococcus lactis found in spinach. Both named folic acid, later found to be identical to vitamin M and vitamin Bc. In 1945 Dr. Tom Spies demonstrated it cured anemia of pregnancy.

*Converted* by liver (in presence of vitamin C) to folinic acid, known also as citrovorum factor, leucovorin.

*Richest food sources* (in μg per 100g) are dried brewer's yeast (2400); soy flour (430); wheat germ (310); wheat bran (260); fresh nuts (110); pig liver (110); green-leaf vegetables (90); legumes (80); oatflakes (60); roasted nuts (57); wheat grains (57); pig kidney (42); whole-wheat bread (39); citrus fruits (peeled) (37); eggs (30); unpolished brown rice (29); white bread (27); fatty fish (26); bananas (22); cheese (9 to 20); root vegetables (15); potatoes (14); dried fruits (14); meats (5 to 12); milk (5). Stored in liver which contains 5 to 15mg per kg.

*Unstable* to oxygen at high temperatures but protected by vitamin C. Unstable to light especially in presence of riboflavin. Leaches into cooking water. Overall losses of 45 per cent can occur in processing and cooking of vegetables, fruits and dairy products.

*Functions* in metabolism of ribonucleic acids (RNA) and deoxyribonucleic acids (DNA) — essential for protein synthesis; formation of blood; transmission of genetic code (hereditary characteristics). Some functions associated with vitamin $B_{12}$. Needed to build up resistance to disease in thymus gland of the new-born and infant.

*Deficiency in man* causes megaloblastic anemia where red blood cells are large and uneven in size and shape with shorter life span. Common in pregnancy.

*Deficiency symptoms* are weakness, fatigue, breathlessness, irritability, sleeplessness eventually giving rise to mild mental symptoms such as forgetfulness and confusion.

*Deficiency in animals* causes anemia and low white blood cell count. Low rate of regeneration of digestive tract, skin, mucous membranes and bone marrow. Low hatchability of turkey eggs.

*Recommended dietary intakes* in the USA are (in μg): babies under one year (45); children 1 to 3 years (100); 4 to 6 years (200); 7 to 10 years (300); all others (400); during pregnancy (800); during lactation (500). WHO recommendation (in μg): babies under 1 year (60); children up to 12 years (100); adolescents 13 to 19 years (200); adult men and women (200); during pregnancy (400); during lactation (300). Intakes not set in the UK.

*Supplementation* limited to 200μg daily in UK for products on general sale.

*Increased requirements* by women taking contraceptive pill, during pregnancy, by the elderly, by alcohol drinkers. By those on the following drugs: methotrexate, pyrimethamine, pentamidime isethionate, trimethoprim, triamterene, phenytoin, isoniazid, aspirin, cholestyramine, primidone. Most require double recommended daily intake but extra requirements when on phenytoin must be monitored since vitamin may neutralize drug.

*During pregnancy* increased intakes necessary (double recommended intake) to prevent birth defects (including neural tube defect causing spina bifida); toxemia; premature birth; hemorrhage following birth, abruptio placentae (premature separation of placenta from uterus); habitual abortion.

*Toxicity* is usually low when taken orally. Occasional reports of loss of appetite, nausea, flatulence, abdominal distension (at 15mg daily). Sleep disturbance, irritability, overactivity. Long-term high dose may cause vitamin $B_{12}$ losses from body.

*Legislative control* of folic acid is not for toxicity reasons but because high intakes may cure anemia symptoms of $B_{12}$ deficiency but not the nerve degeneration that inevitably follows.

*Therapy* with folic acid essential: in all above conditions; in megaloblastic anemia; in schizophrenia, mental deterioration, psychosis; in malabsorption (e.g. sprue) in geriatric patients.

---

**folinic acid,**   citrovorum factor, active form of folic acid produced under the influence of vitamin C in the liver.

---

**Folkers, Karl,**   American scientist who isolated vitamin $B_{12}$ at Merck Laboratories, USA, simultaneously with Lester Smith at Glaxo Laboratories, UK.

---

**food preservatives,**   vitamins C and E are only recognized natural food preservatives but bioflavonoids have some function.

---

**food processing, methods,**   *blanching* — this is required to inactivate enzymes that cause deterioration of food. It always precedes freezing and drying and is a feature of canning. Leaching occurs into the blanching water and the extent of loss depends largely on the time the vegetable is in contact with water. Temperature must be high enough to inactivate the enzymes, i.e., at least 85°C. Garden peas need one minute; sliced beans two minutes; Brussels sprouts from 3.5 to seven minutes depending on size. Temperatures vary from 93 to 99°C and oxidation may contribute to some destruction of the vitamins.

Losses during blanching are estimated to be between 13 and 60 per cent for vitamin C; 2-30 per cent for thiamine; 5-40 per cent for riboflavin.

Carotene losses are less than 1 per cent but these ignore possible transformation into less active forms. Losses due to extraction into water are lessened if the water is consumed. Canning retains all leached vitamins in the liquor so this should not be discarded when the vegetable contents are eaten. Similarly with canned meats. Microwave blanching is reported to cause less damage than steam, and a combination of microwave and hot water treatment is claimed to preserve more vitamins and produce a more palatable product. Fluidized-bed blanching, which is really hot-gas treatment, is claimed to reduce vitamin C and carotene losses. In domestic blanching losses of vitamin C, thiamine and carotene can be prevented by rapid cooling after blanching. Cold air is best to prevent further leaching into water.

*Heat sterilization* — as oxygen is excluded, losses of vitamins are minimal during canning procedures. Thiamine is lost even so, particularly from meat. Best condition to preserve vitamins heating for a short time at high temperature rather than at longer periods at lower temperature.

Losses are less for canned meat and fruit than for vegetables during heat sterilization because the acid conditions are protective. Minor losses only of riboflavin and nicotinic acid occur during heat sterilization of meat. Once the food has been sterilized in cans stability of the vitamins is good. Only 15 per cent of vitamin C is lost after two years' storage of vegetables in cans.

*Freezing* — represents one of the best methods of preserving foods since only the fresh variety is frozen when at the peak of its vitamin content. In frozen meat, most of the vitamins are well preserved but the exudate from thawing can contain appreciable amounts of the water-soluble vitamins. Vegetables must be blanched before freezing so losses are those mentioned under blanching. Similarly during the thawing process the aqueous exudate will contain vitamins so introducing frozen vegetables directly into the heating water will retain them all as long as this water is utilized in the meal. Pyridoxine, pantothenic acid and vitamin E are most affected by deep freezing.

*Irradiation* — causes some losses in vitamins but freeze-drying before treating with ionizing radiation reduces these losses. Most sensitive vitamins are thiamine, riboflavin, vitamin A and vitamin E. Most stable is nicotinic acid.

*Freeze-drying* — this low temperature dehydration is probably the best method of retaining vitamins in the preserved food. It is not, unfortunately, widespread.

*Hot-air drying* — causes variable losses in the different vitamins. Under the most favorable conditions some 10-15 per cent of vitamin C is lost during hot-air drying of vegetables.

*Pressure cooking* — the shortest time required plus the smallest volume of water used reduces vitamin losses compared with conventional boiling. Principal cause of loss is leaching rather than heat but this is limited by volume of water rather than by time of cooking. In many vegetables it has been shown that losses of thiamine in pressure cooking are 25-50 per cent, those in steaming are 50 per cent and those in boiling 75-80 per cent. Vitamin C losses are of the same order but vary amongst different vegetables.

*Microwave heating* — uses high-energy electromagnetic radiation, frequency 2450m Hz, wavelength 12cm, to produce very efficient cooking. Microwaves generate heat throughout the bulk of the food rather than simply applying it to the surface as in a conventional oven. Losses of vitamins may be less than or equal to those associated with conventional cooking methods but they are never more.

General principles to retain the highest vitamin content in foods cooked using domestic methods are:
1.  Use fresh food rather than stored food.
2.  Cook in minimum amount of water.
3.  Minimum cooking at a high temperature is preferable to long cooking at a lower one.
4.  Cooked foods should not be stored before eating except when deep frozen.
5.  Remember that cooking of frozen foods represents the second process they have been through so the whole of the food plus cooking liquids (or thawed exudate) should be utilized. *See also* entries under eggs, fish, meats, milk, vegetables.

---

**food sources,**   in a study carried out in 1980, the percentages of vitamin intakes from various foods in the average UK diet were found to be:

*Thiamine* — 42 per cent derived from bread and cereals; 19 per cent derived from vegetables; 15 per cent derived from meat and organ meats.

*Riboflavin* — 41 per cent derived from milk and milk products; 19 per cent derived from meat and organ meats; 15 per cent derived from bread and cereals.

*Nicotinic acid* — 36 per cent derived from meat and organ meats; 20 per cent derived from cereals and bread; 14 per cent derived from vegetables; 14 per cent derived from milk and milk products.

*Vitamin C* — 50 per cent derived from vegetables; 39 per cent derived from fruit.

*Vitamin A* — 37 per cent derived from meat and organ meats; 24 per cent derived from vegetables; 20 per cent derived from butter and fats; 14 per cent derived from milk and cheeses.

---

**fortification of foods,**   falls into three categories as far as vitamin addition is concerned:

1.   Restoring original vitamin content. In the countries where this is carried out on white flour, restoration is statutory at present but the extent of adding vitamins varies. The recommended additions for white wheat flour (in mg per kg flour) are given in Table 9. Where rice is the staple diet of a country, this also is fortified with vitamins.

**Table 9: Recommended vitamin additions to white wheat flour**

| Country | Thiamine | Riboflavin | Nicotinic acid |
|---|---|---|---|
| Brazil | 4.50 | 2.50 | — |
| Canada | 4.18 | 2.42 | 30.5 |
| Denmark | 5.00 | 5.00 | — |
| Germany | 3.00-4.00 | 1.50-5.00 | 20.0 |
| Great Britain | 2.40 | — | 16.0 |
| Sweden | 2.60-4.00 | 1.20 | 23.0-40.0 |
| Switzerland | 4.18 | 2.53 | 50.0 |
| USA | 4.18 | 2.42-2.53 | 30.5 |
| USSR | 4.00 | 4.00 | 20.0 |

Vitamin C is added to most brands of dehydrated potato to restore that lost during the drying process but this restoration is not obligatory.

Vitamin E is added to some vegetable oils to replace that lost during the refining process. Many cooked cereals have thiamine, riboflavin and nicotinic acid added to them to replace those vitamins lost during refining and processing but this is not obligatory.

2.   Enrichment, where the vitamin is added to give concentrations greater than in the original food. Examples are the addition of vitamin C to fruit juices and drinks; the addition of vitamin A to liquid milk; the addition of all vitamins to dried milk.

3.   Vitaminization — adding vitamins to a food that does not normally

contain them. The process is carried out to ensure that the foods are equal in vitamin content to those for which they are being substituted. One example is margarine, which is produced by hardening of vegetable oils (hard type) or by blending of vegetable oils with partially hardened oils (soft type). As produced margarines are devoid of vitamins A and D so these are added to give the margarine similar content of these vitamins to that of butter. Sometimes vitamin E and polyunsaturated fats are added to increase the intake of these essential nutrients. Addition of vitamins A and D in the USA and UK is statutory; that of other vitamins is not obligatory.

The substitution of expensive animal proteins by cheaper protein is likely to require extensive vitaminization since soy protein is highly refined and processed. To make the two sources of protein equivalent, most vitamins must be added but particularly vitamin $B_{12}$ since this is completely lacking in soy protein.

---

**French beans,** good source of carotene at 400µg per 100g when boiled. Only traces of vitamin E at 0.2mg per 100g. B vitamins present (in mg per 100g) are: thiamine 0.04; riboflavin 0.07; nicotinic acid 0.5; pyridoxine 0.06; pantothenic acid 0.07. Useful source of folic acid at 28µg per 100g but traces only of biotin. Supplies 5mg vitamin C per 100g.

---

**frost bite,** injury to the skin induced by extreme cold and characterized by redness, swelling and pain that can reach deep tissues. In cold climates vitamin C (425mg daily) can help prevent frost bite by maintaining skin temperature.

---

**frozen fries,** contribute B vitamins and vitamin C but when fried, concentrations are increased due to loss of water. B vitamins present (in mg per 100g), in frozen and fried frozen chips respectively, are: thiamine 0.08, 0.09; riboflavin 0.01, 0.02; nicotinic acid 2.1, 2.8; pyridoxine 0.28, 0.39; pantothenic acid — absent. Folic acid levels are 12 and 11µg per 100g respectively. Vitamin C contents are 6 and 4mg per 100g respectively.

---

**frozen peas,** similar vitamin levels to fresh peas and levels of water-soluble vitamins are reduced on boiling to similar degree. Fat-soluble vitamins are unaffected. Carotene levels are unchanged at 0.3mg per 100g and vitamin E levels at 0.9mg per 100g. B vitamin concentrations are (in mg per 100g), frozen raw and boiled respectively: thiamine 0.32, 0.24; riboflavin 0.10, 0.07; nicotinic acid 3.0, 2.4; pyridoxine 0.10, 0.07; pantothenic acid 0.75, 0.32. Good source of folic acid at 78μg per 100g in both frozen raw and boiled peas; biotin levels only 0.5 and 0.4μg per 100g. Vitamin C content reduced from 17 to 13mg per 100g when boiled.

---

**fruit pie filling,**  poor source of vitamins when canned. Those that are present include traces of thiamine, pyridoxine, pantothenic acid and biotin. Traces only of vitamin C. Level of riboflavin is 0.01mg per 100g; folic acid is 1.0μg per 100g.

---

**fruit salad,**  a typical product contains 35 per cent apricots or peaches, 35 per cent pears, 10 per cent cherries, 10 per cent grapes and 10 per cent pineapple. Good source of carotene at 300μg per 100g. B vitamins present are (in mg per 100g): thiamine 0.02; riboflavin 0.01; nicotinic acid 0.3; pyridoxine 0.01; pantothenic acid 0.04. Folic acid level is 4μg per 100g; that of biotin is 0.1μg per 100g. Small amount of vitamin C at 3mg per 100g.

---

**Funk, Casimir,**  Polish chemist who introduced the term "vitamine" in a paper entitled "The Etiology of Deficiency Diseases" in 1911.

---

# G

---

**gallstones,**  cholelithiasis. Over 80 per cent of gallstones are composed of cholesterol, bile pigments and calcium; a further 10 per cent are pure cholesterol. Caused by excess cholesterol in the bile crystallizing into stones. Cholesterol in bile can be reduced with adequate vitamin C intake (up to 1000mg daily).

---

**gammalinolenic acid (GLA),**  usually formed in body from linoleic acid (vitamin F). Substantial amounts found only in oil of evening primrose but some in spirulina. *See* oil of evening primrose.

---

**gamma tocopherol,** *see* E vitamin.

---

**gangrene,** death of a tissue due to failure of arterial blood supply. Late complication of diabetes. May be prevented with adequate intakes of vitamin E throughout life (200-400IU daily). Has been treated with higher intakes of the vitamin (1200IU daily).

Medical advice essential in diabetes because insulin requirements may be reduced at this level of vitamin supplementation.

---

**gastro-intestinal tract,** *see* digestive tract.

---

**gelatin,** provides traces only of all B vitamins except $B_{12}$.

---

**gingivitis,** inflammation of the gums. Has been treated with very high doses of vitamin A (500 000IU) and vitamin E (30IU) daily by injection for six days; then 50 000IU vitamin A three times daily with 200IU vitamin E twice daily for three weeks orally. Complete cure claimed with no relapses.

---

**glandular fever,** also known as infective mononucleosis. Caused by Epstein-Barr virus, one of the herpes type, and characterized by high fever, sore throat and swelling of the lymph glands.

Supplements should include high intake of vitamin C (up to 1500mg daily); high potency vitamin B complex and amino acid L-lysine, 1500mg daily.

---

**glaucoma,** disease of the eye characterized by increased pressure within eyeball causing restricted field of vision, colored halo about lights, lessening of visual power eventually resulting in blindness. Ensure adequate daily intakes of vitamin A (7500IU) and riboflavin (10mg) for good sight. In addition pressure may be reduced with vitamin C (500mg per kg body weight) taken daily over several months.

---

**glossitis,** inflammation of the tongue. Symptom of vitamin $B_{12}$ deficiency. When due to other causes may respond to nicotinamide at doses up to 300mg daily.

---

**glutamic acid,** amino acid, usually supplied by food but can be synthesized within the body. Precursor of gamma-aminobutyric acid (GABA), a natural calming agent produced by the central nervous system. Vitamin $B_6$ essential for GABA synthesis, lack of which causes convulsions in infants.

---

**glutethimide,** hypnotic drug. Prevents absorption of folic acid and prevents conversion of vitamin D to 25-hydroxy vitamin D.

---

**gooseberries,** good source of carotene and vitamin C. Negligible differences between vitamin content of green and ripe gooseberries. Small losses on stewing green variety, with and without sugar. Carotene levels in raw state, stewed without sugar and stewed with sugar respectively (in $\mu$g per 100g) are 180, 150 and 140. Vitamin E levels are respectively (in mg per 100g) 0.4, 0.3, 0.3. B vitamins present (in mg per 100g) are, for raw fruit, stewed without sugar and stewed with sugar respectively: thiamine 0.04, 0.03, 0.03; riboflavin 0.03, 0.03, 0.02; nicotinic acid 0.5, 0.5, 0.3; pyridoxine 0.02, 0.02, 0.02; pantothenic acid 0.15, 0.12, 0.11. Biotin levels are 0.5, 0.4, 0.4$\mu$g per 100g respectively. Vitamin C content is (in mg per 100g) 40 (range 25-50), 31 and 28 respectively for raw fruit, stewed without sugar and stewed with sugar.

*Canned* gooseberries have similar B vitamins and carotene content to stewed, but contain less vitamin C at 24mg per 100g.

---

**gout,** a recurrent acute arthritis of toe and finger joints which results from deposition in the joints and tendons of crystals of sodium urate (uric acid). Has been treated with orotic acid (4g daily for six days) which dissolves uric acid crystals and removes pain and swelling.

---

**grapefruit,** good source of vitamin C with some B vitamins. Traces only of carotene; 0.3mg per 100g vitamin E. In the canned variety vitamin E is reduced to a trace. B vitamins present are (in mg per 100g), for raw (edible part) and canned grapefruit respectively: thiamine 0.05, 0.04; riboflavin 0.02, 0.01; nicotinic acid 0.3, 0.3; pyridoxine 0.03, 0.02; pantothenic acid 0.28, 0.12. Folic acid levels are 12 and 4µg per 100g respectively for raw (edible part) and canned fruit; biotin levels are stable at 1.0µg per 100g. Vitamin C content is 40mg (range 35-45mg) per 100g for the raw edible part and 30mg per 100g for the canned fruit.

---

**grapefruit juice,** freshly expressed variety contains more vitamin C than the canned juice but only minor differences in the B vitamins content. Concentrations of vitamins in sweetened and unsweetened canned juice are identical. Traces of carotene (0.6µg per 100g) in fresh and canned juice. Traces only of vitamin E. B vitamins present are (in mg per 100g), for the fresh and canned juice respectively: thiamine 0.05, 0.04; riboflavin 0.02, 0.01; nicotinic acid 0.30, 0.30; pyridoxine 0.02, 0.01; pantothenic acid 0.16, 0.12. Folic acid levels are 10 and 4µg per 100g respectively; biotin is stable at 1µg per 100g in both. Vitamin C content is 45mg per 100g in the fresh juice, reduced to 29mg per 100g in the canned variety.

---

**grapes,** all varieties have nearly identical amounts of vitamins present. There are traces only of carotene and vitamin E. B vitamins present (in mg per 100g) are: thiamine 0.04; riboflavin 0.02; nicotinic acid 0.3; pyridoxine 0.10; pantothenic acid 0.05. Vitamin C content is 4mg per 100g.

---

**gray hair,** caused by loss of natural pigment. In animals development of gray hair is symptom of pantothenic acid and/or biotin deficiency. No hard evidence that these vitamins prevent graying of hair in man but cases on record where they have restored natural color. PABA deficiency in animals causes premature graying of hair. Color restored with oral PABA but no hard evidence that it does so in man.

---

**greengages,** variety of plums. Poor source of most vitamins that are reduced further by stewing, with and without sugar. Carotene is absent; vitamin E levels (in mg per 100g) for raw fruit, stewed without sugar and stewed with sugar respectively, are 0.7, 0.6, 0.5. B vitamins present are (in mg per 100g), for raw fruit, stewed without sugar and stewed with sugar respectively: thiamine 0.05, 0.04, 0.04; riboflavin 0.03, 0.03, 0.02; nicotinic acid 0.5, 0.4, 0.4; pyridoxine 0.05, 0.03, 0.03; pantothenic acid 0.2, 0.16, 0.14. Only traces of folic acid and biotin are present in both the raw and stewed fruit. Vitamin C content is respectively 3, 3 and 2mg per 100g.

**growth,**  depends on adequate supply of protein, fats, carbohydrates and calories. Transformation of these into growing tissues requires adequate thiamine, riboflavin, pantothenic acid, biotin, vitamin $B_{12}$ and vitamin A during pre-natal and post-natal growth.

**guavas,**  figures available only on canned fruit. Very rich source of vitamin C and useful quantity of carotene present. Carotene content is 100$\mu$g per 100g; vitamin E is virtually absent. B vitamins present are (in mg per 100g): thiamine 0.04; riboflavin 0.03; nicotinic acid 1.0. Vitamin C content is 180mg per 100g. In the raw state this averages 200mg per 100g over the range 20-600mg per 100g.

**gums,**  *see* gingivitis.

**Gyorgy, Paul,**  Professor of Medicine at the University of Pennsylvania, USA, who first isolated vitamin $B_6$ in 1934. First isolated biotin from liver in early 1940s.

# H

**haricot beans,**  virtually devoid of fat-soluble vitamins. B vitamins present include (in mg per 100g): thiamine 0.45; riboflavin 0.13; nicotinic acid 5.9; pyridoxine 0.56; pantothenic acid 0.7. No folic acid or biotin present.

**Hawkins, David,** American doctor who helped introduce megavitamin treatment of mental disease.

---

**hay fever,** a condition characterized by over-secretion of nasal and eye mucous membranes caused by hypersensitivity to pollen. Prevention has been claimed with high doses of vitamin B complex plus extra calcium pantothenate (100mg) and pyridoxine (100mg) in some cases. Treatment includes vitamin C (500mg every 6 hours) which has recognized antihistamine effect. Also claimed that vitamin E (300IU) and bioflavonoids (200mg) daily may bring relief in some people.

---

**hazel nuts,** known also as cob nuts. Kernels are good source of vitamin E and the B vitamins. Vitamin E content is 22.5mg per 100g. B vitamins present are (in mg per 100g): thiamine 0.40; riboflavin appears to be absent; nicotinic acid 3.1; pyridoxine 0.55; pantothenic acid 1.15. Folic acid level is 72$\mu$g per 100g but biotin has not been detected. Traces only of vitamin C present in kernels of hazel nuts.

---

**headache,** a pain or ache anywhere in the head. It is a symptom rather than an illness itself. Causes include: diseases of the eye, nose or throat; sinuses that are blocked or infected; head injury; air pollution or poor ventilation; medicinal drugs; alcohol; tobacco smoking; fever; infections; disturbances of the digestive tract and circulatory system; brain disorders; iron deficiency anemia; low blood sugar; overdose of vitamin A; deficiency of nicotinamide, pyridoxine or calcium pantothenate; allergies.

Treatment depends on underlying cause so professional advice must be sought. Adequate intakes of nicotinamide, pyridoxine, calcium pantothenate and vitamin A may help relieve some headaches.

*Migraine* headaches, *see* migraine.

---

**heart,** edible. Traces only of vitamins A, D and carotene and poor source of vitamin E (0.37-0.70mg per 100g). Good source of B vitamins, supplying the following (in mg per 100g): thiamine 0.21-0.48; riboflavin 0.8-1.5; nicotinic acid 10.6-14.7; pyridoxine 0.11-0.38; pantothenic acid 1.6-3.8. Good source of vitamin $B_{12}$, providing 13-15$\mu$g per 100g. Poor source of folic acid (4$\mu$g) and biotin (3$\mu$g). Vitamin C levels vary from 5 to 11mg per 100g.

---

**heart disease,**  coronary heart disease (CHD) or ischemic heart disease (IHD) are synonymous terms for diseases arising from a failure of the coronary arteries to supply sufficient blood to the heart muscle. These diseases are in most cases associated with atherosclerosis of the coronary arteries. They include myocardial infarction, angina pectoris and sudden death without infarction.

*Myocardial infarction* is death of part of the heart muscle due to failure of blood supply (ischemia). Usually due to blockage of the supplying blood vessel with clot or by fat deposition on the vessel wall. *See* atherosclerosis and blood clot.

*Angina pectoris, see* angina.

*Sudden death* may occur in those who have had myocardial infarction and angina.

Heart disease can be prevented and cured by dietary and supplementary means. Regular vitamin B complex plus high potencies of vitamin E (400-1200IU daily); vitamin C (500-1000mg daily); vitamin $B_6$ (100mg daily); lecithin (15-45g daily); replacement of saturated animal fats in the diet by PUFA (vitamin F) and regular intakes of fish oil containing EPA and DHA may help reduce the chances of heart disease and decrease the possibility of further problems in those who have the complaints.

---

**heavy metal poisoning,**  excess lead, mercury and cadmium in body can be detoxified with high doses of vitamin C (up to 3000mg daily) plus supplementary essential minerals.

---

**hemorrhoids,**  commonly known as piles, characterized by dilated veins of the rectum. Treated with high intakes of bioflavonoids (lemon bioflavonoid complex plus rutin — up to 1000mg daily) plus vitamin C (500mg daily).

---

**hepatitis,**  inflammation of the liver. When due to viral infection can be relieved by very high doses of vitamin C (25-30 grams) for a few days preferably by intravenous injection but also orally by taking 5 grams every four hours. Medical supervision recommended.

High potency multivitamin complex needed to restore vitamins lost from the liver both during and after attack of hepatitis.

---

**herpes simplex,**  cold sores. May respond to daily intakes of essential amino acid L-lysine (0.5-1.5g).

---

**herpes zoster,**  *see* shingles.

---

**Hoffer, Abram,**  American doctor, pioneer of high-potency vitamins in treating schizophrenia in the early 1950s.

---

**honeycomb,**  in the raw state and in jars contains traces only of thiamine and vitamin C. Levels of riboflavin and nicotinic acid are 0.05 and 0.2mg per 100g respectively.

---

**Hopkins, Sir Frederick Gowland,**  British biochemist, who first showed at turn of the century that 'accessory food factors' were essential for health.

---

**horseradish,**  completely devoid of carotene and vitamin E. Levels of B vitamins present (in mg per 100g) are: thiamine 0.05; riboflavin 0.03; nicotinic acid 1.2; pyridoxine 0.15. No other B vitamins present. Excellent source of vitamin C at 120mg per 100g.

---

**hormone replacement therapy (HRT),**  treatment of symptoms of menopause with natural or synthetic female sex hormones. Similar effect on vitamins to those of contraceptive pill. *See* contraceptives, oral. Treated with similar supplements.

---

**hydralazine,**  blood pressure reduction. Enhances excretion of pyridoxine.

---

**hydrocortisone,**  natural corticosteroid hormone present in adrenal glands. *See* corticosteroids.

---

**hydroxocobalamin,**  $B_{12}b$ vitamin.

---

**hyperactivity,** usually occurs in children; characterized by excessive or abnormal activity. Often benefit from high doses of vitamins including nicotinamide (1-3g); pyridoxine (100-300mg); vitamin C (1g); vitamin E (up to 400IU) daily. Constant monitoring essential.

**hypercalcemia,** infantile. High blood level of calcium that may lead to excess calcification of bones, hardening of the arteries and possibly mental retardation. Symptoms of excessive vitamin D intake. May also occur in adults causing deposition of calcium in soft tissues.

**hyperkeratosis,** rough, bumpy skin, once known as "toad skin." Most obvious sign of vitamin A deficiency.

**hypertension,** high blood-pressure. *See* blood-pressure.

# I

**immigrants,** those from Asia are particularly prone to vitamin D deficiency, producing rickets in children and osteomalacia in adults. Reasons not known with certainty but change to Western diet including dairy products, more exposure of skin to sunshine and supplementary vitamin D recommended.

**immune system,** the defence mechanism that the body develops against bacterial and viral infections. Cells responsible arise in thymus gland, spleen and lymphatic system. Impaired by malnutrition and certain vitamin deficiencies. *See* disease resistance.

**impotence,** inability of the male to attain or sustain an erection satisfactorily for normal sexual intercourse. More common in diabetics because they appear to lack ability to convert carotenes to vitamin A which is essential for sex hormone production. Ensure adequate intakes of vitamin A as the preformed vitamin.

---

**inborn errors of metabolism,** a term introduced by Sir Archibald Garrod in 1908 to describe conditions caused by a deficiency of or an error in a single gene. This is the result of a spontaneous or induced mutation in one or both parents and so it becomes part of the genetic make-up of the fetus. These diseases are hence potentially present at the moment of conception. They are completely different from acquired congenital diseases that are due, not to genetic errors, but to defects arising in the uterus.

Several hundred inborn errors of metabolism have been described and there are probably as many more as yet undiscovered. Some of these respond to treatment with a specific vitamin, usually at levels far in excess of normal dietary intakes. The defect is usually in an enzyme that requires the specific vitamin in order to function, or defective absorption of a vitamin, or an inability to transport a vitamin or an inability to convert a vitamin to its active form.

### Thiamine
1. Certain types of maple-syrup urine disease: characterized by delayed nervous system development. Due to defective enzyme that requires thiamine pyrophosphate as coenzyme. Responds to 10mg thiamine daily.
2. Lactic acidosis: characterized by persistent low blood sugar and acidosis due to accumulation of lactic acid. Deficient enzyme is pyruvate carboxylase. Responds to 10mg thiamine daily.

### Nicotinamide
1. Hartnup disease: characterized by intermittent skin rash and mental disturbance, symptoms similar to pellagra. Appears partly due to impaired intestinal absorption of tryptophane, an amino acid that is a precursor of nicotinamide. Skin and mental symptoms respond to 100mg of nicotinamide daily.
2. Hydroxykynureninuria: symptoms are mild, mental deficiency; short stature; rash on buttocks and ulceration of the mouth. Responds to 100mg of nicotinamide daily.

### Pyridoxine
1. Infantile convulsions: symptoms are convulsions, excessive irritability,

and acute sense of hearing immediately after birth. Responds to 10mg pyridoxine daily by mouth. Treatment must continue for many years.

2.  Cystathioninuria: symptoms are mental retardation and congenital defects with an increased tendency to bleed. Pituitary gland abnormalities. Due to large amounts of amino acid cystathionine in blood and urine because body cannot metabolize it. Pyridoxal phosphate is coenzyme for the enzyme cystathioninase which is defective. Responds to high doses (more than 10mg per day) of pyridoxine.

3.  Hypochromic anemia: anemia with high blood serum iron and increased iron stores. Due to defective enzyme delta-aminolaevulinic acid synthetase. Usually, but not always, responds to large doses of pyridoxine at levels of 20-100mg per day.

4.  Homocystinuria: characterized by an excessive excretion of the amino acid homocystine in the urine. Some cases respond to very large doses of pyridoxine at levels of 200-500mg per day.

5.  Xanthurenic aciduria: characterized by excessive excretion of xanthurenic acid after high tryptophane meal. Symptoms are defective mental states. Sometimes responds to large doses, up to 200mg per day, of pyridoxine.

## Biotin

Propionic acidemia: acidosis in the new-born due to accumulation of propionic acid in the blood. Caused by a defect in the enzyme propionyl — CoA carboxylase which requires biotin. Responds well to 10mg biotin daily.

## Folic acid

1.  Congenital defect in folate absorption: deficiency of folic acid caused by a defect in its absorption from the food and inability to transport the vitamin. Characterized by anemia; mental retardation; seizures; involuntary movement; impairment of voluntary movement. Anemia responds to doses of folic acid of 40mg per day but fits may not respond.

2.  Formimino-transferase enzyme deficiency: symptoms are retarded mental and physical development; blood shows increased folic acid level. Condition involves vitamin but does not respond to it.

## Vitamin $B_{12}$

1.  Malabsorption of the vitamin not due to lack of intrinsic factor. Characterized by megaloblastic anemia that responds only to injections of vitamin $B_{12}$.

2.  Congenital lack of intrinsic factor. Occurs early in life and is due to

non-production of intrinsic factor for reasons unknown. Responds completely to injections of vitamin $B_{12}$.

3.   Megaloblastic anemia due to lack of specific transport protein (transcobalamin II) of vitamin $B_{12}$ in the blood. Usually occurs in newborn. Responds to injections of 1mg vitamin $B_{12}$ on regular and prolonged basis.

4.   Lack of other specific protein (transcobalamin I) carrier of vitamin $B_{12}$ in the blood. Characterized by low vitamin $B_{12}$ blood levels but no other signs of deficiency.

5.   Methylmalonicaciduria: acidosis in the blood of the new-born. Large amounts of methylmalonic acid in the urine. Due to inability to form the coenzyme form of vitamin $B_{12}$ called 5'-Deoxyadenosyl cobalamin. Responds to frequent injections of high-dose (1mg) vitamin $B_{12}$ or the coenzyme $B_{12}$ itself.

### Vitamin A

The condition is due to an inability to convert carotene to vitamin A. One case only has been described and the symptoms include night blindness, dry eyes (Bitots spots), low blood plasma vitamin A with high blood carotene level. Can be treated by administration of preformed vitamin A.

### Vitamin D

1.   Hereditary vitamin D-resistant rickets with hypophosphatemia: low phosphate levels in the blood but calcium levels are normal. Primary abnormality is inability to reabsorb phosphate in the kidney. Main disease is rickets or osteomalacia and dwarfism. Treatment is very high doses of vitamin daily (2.5mg or 100 000IU) but this can cause intoxication. May respond better to high oral intakes of phosphate.

2.   Fanconi's Syndrome: rickets or osteomalacia with low blood phosphate resistant to normal vitamin D intakes. Due to an inability of the kidneys to acidify urine resulting also in low blood potassium levels. Accumulation of the amino acid cystine in the blood and excessive excretion of amino acids in the urine. May respond to massive doses of vitamin D but possible toxic effects must be monitored.

3.   Primary renal tubular acidosis: usually affects females in late childhood. Characterized by chronic acidosis, osteomalacia, calcium deposits in the kidneys, stones in the kidneys. Increased excretion of calcium and phosphate in the urine leading to low blood levels of the minerals. Treatment of the acidosis is with citrate and in some cases vitamin D is required but it is not standard therapy.

**indomethacin,** anti-arthritic drug. Impairs vitamin C and thiamine utilization.

**inositol,** water-soluble member of vitamin B complex. Not regarded as true vitamin in man since body can synthesize it. High concentration in brain and in stomach, kidney, spleen, liver and heart. Also known as bios I; myo-inositol; meso-inositol; lipotropic factor. Phytic acid is inositol hexaphosphoric acid. Present in supplements as inositol; inositol niacinate; lecithin. Colorless, crystalline substance.

*Richest food sources* (in mg per 100g) are: lecithin granules (2857); beef heart (1600); desiccated liver (1100); wheat germ (690); lecithin oil (360); liver (340); brown rice (330); oatflakes (320); beef steak (260); citrus fruits, peeled (210); wheat grains (190); nuts (180); molasses (180); legumes (160); bananas (120); whole-wheat bread (100); green-leaf vegetables (100); white bread (75); soy flour (70); chicken, corn, root vegetables, dried brewer's yeast (all 50).

*Present* in cereals and vegetables as phytic acid.

*Produced* from glucose by intestinal bacteria.

*Stable* to cooking methods and food processing.

*Functions* as lipotropic factor that prevents accumulation of fats in liver and other organs; as mild anti-anxiety agent; to maintain healthy hair; to control blood cholesterol level.

*Deficiency in man* causes no specific disease or symptoms apart from those associated with loss of functions mentioned above.

*Deficiency in animals* causes fatty liver; loss of hair; muscular dystrophy.

*Recommended dietary intakes* have not been set by any authority. Normal daily intake probably between 300mg and 1000mg from diet. Also synthesized by intestinal bacteria.

*Toxicity* — no reports of toxic effects even with very high doses. As phytic acid it may immobilize some minerals but no effect on vitamin absorption.

*Therapy* with inositol beneficial in reducing blood cholesterol level; in restoring healthy hair; has mild inhibiting effect on cancer; with vitamin E has been used to treat mild nerve damage in some forms of muscular dystrophy; as anti-anxiety agent; in treating irritability; in treating schizophrenia.

**insect repellant,** thiamine in daily doses of 75-100mg acts in those who are prone to insect bites, probably because odor of vitamin in skin is repugnant to insects.

---

**international units (IU),**  means of expressing vitamins in terms of biological activity. Now mainly superseded by expressing them as weight (milligrams or micrograms). Only three left that are still measured in units:

Vitamin A, one IU = 0.30 micrograms retinol
One IU beta carotene = 0.10 micrograms retinol
Vitamin D, one IU = 0.025 micrograms
Vitamin E, one IU = 1.0 milligram dl-alpha tocopheryl acetate *or* 0.91mg dl-alpha tocopherol *or* 0.74mg d-alpha tocopheryl acetate *or* 0.67 d-alpha tocopherol *or* 1.12mg dl-alpha tocopheryl succinate *or* 0.83mg d-alpha tocopheryl succinate.

Other vitamins that were expressed once in international units are:

thiamine hydrochloride, one IU = 3 micrograms
pantothenic acid, one IU = 13.33 micrograms
vitamin C, one IU = 50 micrograms

---

**intestinal surgery,**  post-operative nausea and distension reduced by 250mg calcium pantothenate daily. Vitamin C (1000mg per day) before and after operation will accelerate healing process.

---

**intrinsic factor,**  specific protein secreted by the stomach that forms a complex with vitamin $B_{12}$ in the diet. Complex is then absorbed in the ileum, the lower part of the small intestine. Lack of intrinsic factor gives rise to pernicious anemia because $B_{12}$ in diet cannot be absorbed. Factor may also be deficient in those who have had stomach or part of it removed.

  Giving intrinsic factor with vitamin $B_{12}$ may help absorb the vitamin but eventually the factor may no longer be effective as it is derived from animals. No more than 8 micrograms of oral dose of vitamin $B_{12}$ absorbed by intrinsic factor mechanism at one time.

---

**iron,**  mineral required for formation of hemoglobin, the oxygen-carrying factor of blood. Absorption from food and supplements more efficient in presence of vitamin C. Vitamin E destroyed only by ferric form not more acceptable ferrous form.

**isoniazid,**  anti-tuberculosis drug. Enhances excretion of pyridoxine.

**isotretinoin,**  isomer of retinoic acid, less toxic than tretinoin and given orally.

**IUD,**  intra-uterine contraceptive device or coil. *See* contraceptives.

# J

**jam,**  good source of vitamin C in whole-fruit jam at 10mg per 100g; black currant jam contains 24mg per 100g. Traces only of carotene, vitamin E, thiamine, riboflavin, nicotinic acid, pyridoxine, folic acid, pantothenic acid and biotin.

**Jansen, B. C. P.,**  Dutch doctor who with Dr. W. F. Donath first isolated vitamin $B_1$ from rice polishings in 1926.

**jaundice,**  obstructive. Yellow skin due to excessive bile pigments overflowing from liver because of bile duct blockage. Causes deficient absorption of fat soluble vitamins, particularly vitamin K, which is given by injection. Water-solubilized vitamin E required.

# K

**K,** fat-soluble vitamin. Abbreviation for koagulations — vitamin (Danish). Occurs naturally in foods as vitamin $K_1$, also known as phytomenadione, phylloquinone, phytylmenaquinone, anti-hemorrhagic vitamin. Only one vitamin $K_1$. Also available as vitamin $K_2$ produced by bacteria either in intestine or in fermentations as in putrefying food. $K_2$ is a group of vitamins known as multiprenyl-menaquinones with carbon chains containing from 20 to 65 carbon atoms. Abbreviated to menaquinone-4 to menaquinone-13 (numbers refer to isoprenyl units, each containing 5 carbon atoms). Vitamins $K_2$ only 75 per cent activity of $K_1$. Synthetic vitamin known as $K_3$ or menadione or menaphthone has twice activity of $K_1$. Present in supplements as acetomenaphthone, a synthetic derivative. $K_1$ isolated from alfalfa by Dr. Henrik Dam in 1935 at University of Frieberg. $K_2$ isolated from decayed fishmeal by Dr. Edward Daisy of St Louis University, USA, in 1939.

*Richest food sources* (in µg per 100g) are: cauliflower (3600); Brussels sprouts (800); broccoli (800); lettuce (700); spinach (600); pig liver (600); cabbage (400); tomatoes (400); string beans (290); beef liver (200); lean meat (100); potatoes (80); peas (30); cow's milk (20).

Substantial amounts of $K_2$ produced by intestinal bacterial synthesis. Probably at least 50 per cent of daily intake.

*Destroyed* by acids, alkalis, oxidizing agents, light and ultra-violet irradiation, hence most survives domestic cooking methods. Some losses in commercial processing including deep-freezing.

*Functions* solely in blood coagulation or clotting, not directly but essential for synthesis of four specific proteins that act in coagulation process.

*Deficiency* reduces coagulability of blood leading to excessive bleeding and hemorrhage.

*Deficiency symptoms* appear in hemorrhagic disease of the new-born and are characterized as bleeding from the stomach, the intestine, umbilical stump and operation sites on second or third day after birth.

*Deficiency induced* in new-born because of poor transfer across placenta, low levels in human breast milk, sterile intestine with no bacteria. In adults malabsorption of fats due to lack of bile salts as in biliary obstruction; as a consequence of sprue; in celiac disease; surgical removal of intestine; after prolonged liquid paraffin ingestion; with liver complaints such as viral hepatitis, cirrhosis and cancer. Deficiency also caused by destruction of intestinal bacteria by antibiotics.

*Recommended dietary intakes* have not been set by any authority, mainly because of widespread distribution in food, intestinal bacterial synthesis, lack of evidence of widespread deficiency. Different studies suggest daily requirement can vary from 40µg per day to 30µg per kg body weight. Variations probably due to different rates of bacterial synthesis and efficiency of absorption.

*Increased dietary intakes* needed in new-born babies; in anyone with malabsorption disease; in those with biliary obstruction; in those with liver disease; in those taking antibiotics for long periods; on prolonged liquid paraffin ingestion; in overdose of anticoagulant drugs.

*Toxicity* effects have not been reported.

*Therapy* has been confined to treating hemorrhagic disease of the new-born; in overcoming the inability to absorb the vitamin for various reasons; in overcoming the effects of antibiotics on the intestinal bacteria; in treating overdose of the anticoagulant drug. *Anticoagulant* drugs function by neutralizing the effect of vitamin K. These drugs are warfarin and dicoumarol.

---

**kanamycin,**   antibiotic. Prevents absorption of vitamins K and $B_{12}$.

---

**keratinization,**   formation of hard, dry, scaly cells in place of normal healthy cells in wet surfaces of the body, particularly around eyes, mouth and lining of reproductive tract. Symptom of vitamin A deficiency.

---

**kidney,**   edible. Good source of vitamin A (from 140 to 250µg per 100g) but negligible quantities of carotene and vitamin D. Supplies useful quantities of B vitamins, particularly vitamin $B_{12}$, at levels of (in mg per 100g): thiamine 0.19-0.56; riboflavin 1.9-2.3; nicotinic acid 11.0-14.9; pyridoxine 0.25-0.32; pantothenic acid 2.4-5.1; vitamin $B_{12}$ 0.015-0.079; folic acid 0.042-0.079; biotin 0.024-0.053. Vitamin C levels are from 9 to 14mg per 100g.

---

**kidney stones,**   also known as renal stones, renal calculi or urinary calculi. Common causes of back pain, obstruction and secondary infection. Over 90 per cent are composed of calcium salts.

*Therapy* and prevention involves pyridoxine (up to 100mg daily) plus magnesium (300mg daily) as amino acid chelate to dissolve calcium and prevent its precipitation.

---

**Klenner, Frederick R.,**  American doctor who has published many research papers on treatment of disease with vitamin C.

---

**Krebs, E. T.,**  American biochemist who with his son isolated pangamic acid ($B_{15}$) and laetrile ($B_{17}$) from apricot kernels in the early 1950s.

---

**Kuhn, R.,**  German doctor who first isolated vitamin $B_2$ from milk in 1928.

---

# L

---

**lactoflavin(e),**  $B_2$ vitamin.

---

**laetrile,**  water-soluble factor present in vitamin B complex. Also known as amygdalin, $B_{17}$, vitamin $B_{17}$ (incorrectly); full name laevo-mandelonitrile-beta-glucuronoside. First isolated from apricot kernels in early 1950s by father and son team of Drs. E. T. Krebs and E. T. Krebs Jr. White crystalline powder. Present in supplements as laetrile.

*Richest sources* are apricot pits (average 5mg per pit); peach pits; apple seeds; bitter almonds; cherry pits; plum pits; lime seeds; pear seeds; some grasses; some berries (figures not known).

*Unstable* to heat so pits are usually eaten raw.

*Functions* as source of organic cyanide. Cancer cells believed to convert organic cyanide to inorganic cyanide but unable to detoxify it. Hence inorganic cyanide specifically destroys cancer cells.

*Deficiency in man* has not been reported.

*Deficiency in animals* has not been reported.

*Recommended dietary intakes* not set by any authority.

*Toxicity* is due entirely to cyanide content.

*Toxic symptoms* are cold sweats, headaches, nausea, lethargy, breathlessness, blue lips, low blood pressure — all associated with excess cyanide. Injectable laetrile less toxic than oral dosing.

*Controlled* by DHSS and available only on prescription.

*Therapy* with laetrile confined to cancer but benefits very controversial. Injectable preparation preferred but regarded as only part of holistic approach.

---

**lamb,** all cuts when cooked supply only traces of vitamins A, D and carotene. Vitamin E ranges from 0.04 to 0.18mg per 100g. Poor source of folic acid and biotin. Other B vitamins present (in mg per 100g) are in the range: thiamine 0.06-0.15; riboflavin 0.13-0.38; nicotinic acid 7.5-13.1; pyridoxine 0.11-0.25; pantothenic acid 0.3-0.7; (in $\mu$g per 100g) vitamin $B_{12}$ 1-2; folic acid 2-4.

Higher potencies associated with leaner cuts. Completely devoid of vitamin C. *See also* Meats: Cooking losses.

---

**lard,** pork fat. Devoid of carotene and vitamin C. Traces only of vitamins A and D and of all the B vitamins.

---

**laverbread,** made from edible seaweed. Contains no carotene. Supplies 1.1mg vitamin E per 100g. Levels of B vitamins present (in mg per 100g) are: thiamine 0.03; riboflavin 0.10; nicotinic acid 1.1. No other B vitamins present apart from folic acid at 47$\mu$g per 100g. Vitamin C content is 5mg per 100g.

---

**learning disabilities,** inability to learn and concentrate in children and adolescents. Usually associated with hyperactivity. Megavitamin therapy, *see* hyperactivity.

---

**lecithin,** a complex mixture of phospholipids combined with vegetable oils, fatty acids and sugars. Refined grades of lecithin may contain these ingredients in varying proportions and combinations. Consistency varies from liquid lecithin to solid granules depending upon the free fatty acid

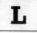 

and oil content. Color varies from light yellow to brown depending upon source, crop variation and whether it has been bleached. It is odorless or with a slight nut-like odor and a bland taste.

Lecithin can only be called such when it contains at least 50 per cent phospholipids or phosphatides. At this level it is a brown liquid that is usually presented in soft gelatine capsules and tablets.

Precipitation of this oil with acetone produces a solid containing up to 98 per cent phosphatides. This is presented as light yellow granules and is the purest lecithin available. The most important phosphatides from a nutritional viewpoint are phosphatidyl choline, phosphatidyl inositol and phosphatidyl ethanolamine.

Lecithin occurs in all animals and vegetable cells. In human beings highest concentrations are in brain, liver, kidneys and bone marrow.

*Richest food sources* (in mg per 100g) are: liver (850); meats (450-750); trout (580); eggs (350); butter (150) in animal foods. In vegetables they are: wheat (2820); soy bean (1480); peanuts (1113); corn (953); oats (650); polished rice (580).

*Daily requirement* not set because body capable of making it.

*Functions* as lipotropic agent in keeping fats in suspension in blood; preventing fatty infiltration of liver and other vital organs; as constituent of fatty membranes; as constituent of myelin sheath around nerves; as provider of choline, needed for nerve impulse transmission; as provider of inositol.

Lecithins from vegetable sources are preferred because the fatty acids in them are PUFA. Those from animal sources tend to contain saturated and mono-unsaturated fatty acids.

*Pure lecithin* granules contain per 5g: 2.86g PUFA; 1.11g phosphatidyl choline; 0.69g phosphatidyl inositol; 0.71g choline; 0.14g inositol and provide 43 calories. Lecithin oil (as capsules) provides half these quantities.

*Toxicity* not reported with lecithin.

*Therapy* with lecithin has given benefit in reducing high blood-pressure; in reducing blood cholesterol levels; in reducing blood fat levels; in preventing and solubilizing gallstones; in treating atherosclerosis; in treating arteriosclerosis; as preventative treatment in angina and following heart attacks and strokes; in treating Alzheimer's disease and senile dementia.

---

**leeks,** the bulbs contain 40μg carotene per 100g in both raw and boiled vegetables; leaves are much richer, supplying 2000μg per 100g. Vitamin E level is 0.8mg per 100g. All levels of B vitamins reduced on boiling. Concentrations (in mg per 100g), for raw and boiled respectively, are:

thiamine 0.10, 0.07; riboflavin 0.05, 0.03; nicotinic acid 0.9, 0.7; pyridoxine 0.25, 0.15; pantothenic acid 0.12, 0.10. Biotin levels are 1.4 and 1.0µg per 100g respectively; folic acid present in boiled variety is 7.0µg per 100g.

**leg cramps,** *see* cramps.

**lemon curd,** homemade variety is richer source of vitamins than commercial starch-based product. Vitamin A levels for commercial and homemade curd (in µg per 100g) are respectively 10 and 130. The homemade variety also provides 60µg carotene per 100g and 0.55µg vitamin D per 100g. Levels of B vitamins, for commercial and homemade curd (in mg per 100g) respectively, are: thiamine, trace, 0.02; riboflavin, trace, 0.12; nicotinic acid 0.1, 1.0; pyridoxine, trace, 0.3; pantothenic acid 0.10, 0.49. Folic acid levels are a trace and 4µg per 100g respectively; biotin levels are 1 and 7µg per 100g. Traces of vitamin $B_{12}$ in both products. Vitamin C contents are a trace and 8mg per 100g respectively for commercial and homemade curds.

**lemonade,** commercially-bottled variety contributes traces only of carotene, vitamin E, thiamine, riboflavin, nicotinic acid, pyridoxine, pantothenic acid, folic acid and biotin. Traces also of vitamin C but this may be increased in some brands to 5-15mg per 100g when fortified.

**lemons,** good source of vitamin C plus some B vitamins. Edible part of lemon fruit has higher levels of vitamins than freshly expressed juice. Traces only of carotene and vitamin E. B vitamins present are (in mg per 100g), for edible fruit and fresh juice respectively: thiamine 0.05, 0.02; riboflavin 0.04, 0.01; nicotinic acid 0.3, 0.1; pyridoxine 0.11, 0.15; pantothenic acid 0.23, 0.10. Folic acid cannot be measured in whole fruit but fresh juice contains 7µg per 100g. Biotin levels are 0.5 and 0.3µg per 100g respectively for fruit and juice. Vitamin C content of whole lemons is 80mg per 100g; fresh juice contains 50mg (range 40-60mg) per 100g.

**lentils,** good source of carotene and B vitamins in raw state but substantial losses on splitting and boiling. Carotene levels (in µg per 100g) in raw and boiled states are 60 and 20 respectively. Levels of B vitamins (in mg per 100g), raw figures first, are: thiamine 0.50, 0.11; riboflavin 0.04, 0.03; nicotinic acid 5.8, 1.6; pyridoxine 0.60, 0.11; pantothenic acid 1.36, 0.31. Folic acid level drops from 35 to 5μg per 100g on boiling. Biotin not detected. Negligible amounts of vitamin C present.

**lettuce,** useful source of carotene, vitamin E and B vitamins. Carotene content averages 1.0mg per 100g but outer green leaves may contain up to fifty times as much carotene as inner white ones. Vitamin E level is 1.2mg per 100g. Contents of B vitamins (in mg per 100g) are: thiamine 0.07; riboflavin 0.08; nicotinic acid 0.4; pyridoxine 0.07; pantothenic acid 0.20. Folic acid content is 34μg per 100g; biotin only 0.7μg. Good source of vitamin C at average 15mg per 100g.

**leucocytes,** white blood cells. Function as phagocytes that engulf invading micro-organisms. Efficiency depends upon mobility of the leucocytes and on their antimicrobial action. Both factors require adequate vitamin C concentration in leucocytes. Those with low resistance to infection need up to 3 grams vitamin C daily to ensure adequate levels.

Lymphocytes are white blood cells that produce antibodies to neutralize invading organisms. Vitamin C in lymphocytes essential for antibody production. Children with deficient lymphocytes exhibit normal defence response to infection with one gram of vitamin C daily.

**lime juice cordial,** in undiluted form provides traces only of carotene, vitamin E, thiamine, riboflavin, nicotinic acid, pyridoxine, pantothenic acid, folic acid, biotin and vitamin C.

**limes,** identical vitamin content to lemons, apart from vitamin C. Vitamin C levels are 35mg per 100g fruit and 25mg per 100g in fresh juice.

**Lind, James,** Scottish naval surgeon, credited with the first known controlled clinical trial, reported in 1753, that showed that citrus fruits were able to prevent and cure the disease scurvy.

**lipids,** general term for all fatty substances including fats, oils, phospholipids (lecithin), cholesterol, triglycerides, fatty acids. *See* under individual headings.

---

**lipoic acid,**   known also as thioctic acid. Regarded as vitamin for bacteria, protozoa, plants and some animals. Essential for pyruvate oxidation in these species. Not regarded as essential in man but has been used as therapy in treatment of liver disease and in poisoning by non-edible mushrooms.

---

**liqueurs,**   contain traces of all B vitamins, including vitamin $B_{12}$.
*Advocaat* provides traces of vitamin D also because of egg content.

---

**liquid paraffin,**   anti-constipation agent. Prevents absorption of vitamins A, D, E and K and carotenes.

---

**liver,**   largest gland in the body forming one-fortieth of body weight.
*Storage* depot for vitamins A, D, riboflavin, pantothenic acid, biotin, folic acid, pyridoxine, vitamin $B_{12}$ and vitamin C. Contains sufficient vitamin A, D and $B_{12}$ to last 6 months to 2 years in well-fed person. Other vitamins must be replenished regularly every day or so.
*Site* for activation of all vitamins, i.e., conversion of thiamine, riboflavin, nicotinamide, pyridoxine, pantothenic acid, biotin into phosphate complexes; conversion of folic acid to folinic acid; conversion of vitamin $B_{12}$ into its coenzyme forms; conversion of vitamin D into 25-hydroxy vitamin D; conversion of vitamin A into retinoic acid. All these transformations essential before vitamins can perform metabolic functions. *Site* for synthesis of choline and inositol and further incorporation into lecithin. *Site* for conversion of cholesterol into bile salts, dependent on vitamin C. *Site* for production of proteins needed for blood clotting, dependent upon vitamin K.
*Diseases of liver* can cause excessive loss of all vitamins but especially the B complex; can prevent uptake of vitamins by the liver; can reduce efficiency of activation of vitamins into metabolic forms.
*Alcohol* and some medicinal drugs can have similar effects on vitamins.
*Fatty liver* due to deficiency of choline and inositol.

---

**liver,**   edible. From all sources supplies large quantities of vitamin A and carotene and provides some vitamins D and E. Quantities are (in mg per 100g): vitamin A 9.3-20.6; carotene 0.1-1.54; vitamin E 0.24-0.50. Vitamin D ranges from 1.7 to 4.4μg per 100g.

Good source of all B vitamins and liver has the highest vitamin $B_{12}$ and folic acid contents of any animal product. Concentrations are (in mg per 100g): thiamine 0.18-0.37; riboflavin 1.7-4.4; nicotinic acid 14.3-21.4; pyridoxine 0.40-0.83; pantothenic acid 4.6-8.8; vitamin $B_{12}$ 0.025-0.111; folic acid 0.11-0.50; biotin 0.027-0.17.

Vitamin C concentrations are from 10 to 23mg per 100g.

---

**LLD factor,**   *see* $B_{12}$ vitamin.

---

**loganberries,**   good source of vitamin C with some carotene and B vitamins present. Carotene contents (in μg per 100g) of raw fruit, stewed without sugar and stewed with sugar are 80, 75 and 70 respectively; vitamin E is present at concentrations of 0.3mg per 100g in each variety. B vitamins present (in mg per 100g) in raw fruit, stewed without sugar and stewed with sugar respectively, are: thiamine 0.02, 0.02, 0.02; riboflavin 0.03, 0.03, 0.03; nicotinic acid 0.6, 0.6, 0.4; pyridoxine 0.06, 0.05, 0.05; pantothenic acid 0.24, 0.20, 0.18. Folic acid and biotin are virtually absent. Vitamin C contents are (in mg per 100g) 35, 29 and 26 respectively for the three varieties.

*Canned* loganberries have slightly reduced vitamin levels from the stewed fruit. The figures are (in mg per 100g): thiamine 0.01; riboflavin 0.02; nicotinic acid 0.4; pyridoxine 0.04; pantothenic acid 0.17; vitamin C 25.

---

**losses in food processing,**   the term food processing includes domestic cooking techniques as well as those used in the food manufacturing industry. Losses of nutrients, particularly vitamins, may be summed up as follows:

1.   Some loss of vitamins is inevitable but, except for the examples quoted below, most losses are small.

2.   Manufacturing losses, when they occur, are sometimes comparable to those in domestic cooking losses.

3.   When foods are further cooked at home, losses of vitamins are additional to those incurred during the manufacturing process.

4.   It is easier and more convenient to recover vitamins lost during

domestic cooking (e.g. by utilizing cooking water) than those lost in factory processing.

5.    The importance of the losses in a particular food must be considered in relation to the whole diet. When the food makes only a small contribution to the intake of vitamins, processing losses may not be significant. However, losses from foods that make up a significant part of the diet, like milk and cereal products for babies and cereals in some countries, can cause serious deficiencies in those relying on such diets.

6.    Some processing methods confer nutritional advantages on the vitamin content of food, e.g. trypsin inhibitors in some vegetables are destroyed by cooking and nicotinic acid is liberated from its inactive bound form by the cooking of cereals.

7.    Under-processing of some foods may not destroy harmful micro-organisms in those foods. Processing can improve appearance and flavor of some foods and allow preservation for all-round-the-year availability. The ideal conditions of food processing allow these advantages with only minimal destruction and loss of vitamins.

*Vitamin A* — Both vitamin A and carotene are insoluble in water so do not suffer from losses through extraction into processing and cooking water. The main destructive agent is oxygen but in foods they tend to be protected by natural antioxidants like vitamin E.

Destruction of vitamin A and carotenes is accelerated by peroxides and free radicals formed from accompanying fats, particularly those of the polyunsaturated variety. Peroxides and free radicals in turn are formed by high temperatures and oxygen and promoted by light, traces of iron and the presence of copper.

Boiling water destroys 16 per cent of the vitamin A in margarine in 30 minutes, 40 per cent in one hour and 70 per cent in two hours. Frying at 200°C destroys 40 per cent of the vitamin A in margarine in five minutes, 60 per cent in ten minutes and 70 per cent in fifteen minutes. Braising liver causes up to 10 per cent loss of vitamin A.

Earlier reports of complete stability of carotene in canned foods are now regarded as unreliable as only total carotenoids were measured. Canning converts some of the carotene with 100 per cent activity into another form with only 38 per cent activity. Green vegetables are thus shown to lose 15-20 per cent of their vitamin A activity; yellow vegetables lose 30-25 per cent of their activity after freezing or canning followed by further cooking. There is no difference, despite varying temperatures and cooking times, between commercial canning, pressure cooking and boiling or baking of these vegetables.

Vitamin A (as carotene) losses in vegetables and fruits range from 10-20 per cent under controlled, mild conditions of drying to virtual complete destruction in traditional open-air drying. Losses of vitamin A and carotene also occur on storage in accordance with the figures shown in Table 10.

**Table 10: Losses of vitamin A and carotene in stored foods**

| Food | Vitamin A | | | Carotene | | |
|---|---|---|---|---|---|---|
| | Months stored | Temp. °C | Percentage loss | Months stored | Temp. °C | Percentage loss |
| Butter | 12 | 5 | 0-30 | — | — | — |
| | 5 | 28 | 35 | — | — | — |
| Margarine | 6 | 5 | 0-10 | 6 | 5 | 0 |
| | 6 | 23 | 0-20 | 6 | 23 | 10 |
| Skimmed milk powder | 3 | 37 | 0-5 | — | — | — |
| | 12 | 23 | 10-30 | — | — | — |
| Fortified lard | — | — | — | 6 | 5 | 0 |
| | | | | 6 | 23 | 0 |
| Dried egg-yolk | — | — | — | 3 | 37 | 5 |
| | | | | 12 | 23 | 20 |
| Fortified cereal | 6 | 23 | 20 | — | — | — |
| Fortified potato chips | 2 | 23 | 0 | — | — | — |
| Carbonated beverage | — | — | — | 2 | 30 | 5 |
| Canned juice | — | — | — | 12 | 23 | 0-15 |

*Thiamine* — apart from vitamin C, thiamine is the least stable of the vitamins. Stable only under acid conditions, destruction is catalysed by copper. Completely inactivated by sulphur dioxide, a widespread preservative added to foods, e.g. mince containing sulphur dioxide loses 90 per cent of its thiamine in 48 hours. Protein and amino acids protect thiamine in foods, and starch assists by absorbing the vitamin. Cereals are added to pork to help stabilize thiamine in cooked meats.

Principal losses of thiamine are due to its water solubility; the more finely ground the food the greater the loss. Chopped and minced foods can lose from 20-70 per cent of their thiamine which can be recovered by eating the extracted liquors. Cooking meat at temperatures up to 150°C causes no destruction of the vitamin but considerable losses into the exuded juices. At temperatures of 200°C, 20 per cent of the thiamine is destroyed.

The vitamin is not lost by leaching when boiling rice in distilled water but 8-10 per cent is lost in tap water and 36 per cent is lost in well water, indicating the effects of alkalinity. Baking processes cause 15-25 per cent loss of the vitamin but adding baking powder increases it to 50 per cent.

Amongst vegetables, only potatoes contribute significant amounts of thiamine (about 15 per cent of the daily intakes) to the diet. Ready-peeled potatoes and potato chips are kept white by adding sulphite solution causing 55 per cent destruction of the vitamin present. Further frying results in 10 per cent additional loss from unpreserved variety and 20 per cent from the vegetable soaked in sulphite solution. Commercial processing causes 24 per cent losses in potatoes dipped in sulphite solution after three days' storage at 5°C; further losses on frying can be 30 per cent.

**Table 11: Losses of thiamine during cooking**

| Meat | Cooking method | Percentage loss |
| --- | --- | --- |
| Beef | roast | 40-60 |
| | broiled | 50 |
| | stewed | 50-70 |
| | fried | 0-45 |
| | braised | 40-45 |
| | canned | 80 |
| Pork | braised | 20-30 |
| | roast | 30-40 |
| Ham | baked | 50 |
| | fried | 50 |
| | broiled | 20 |
| | canned | 50-60 |
| Chop | braised | 15 |
| Bacon | fried | 80 |
| Mutton | broiled chop | 30-40 |
| | roast leg | 40-50 |
| | stewed lamb | 50 |
| Poultry | roast chicken, turkey | 30-45 |
| Fish | fried | 40 |

Bread baking gives rise to losses of 15-30 per cent of thiamine contained in the flour (mainly in the crust) but it is stable in the finished loaf. Toasting of bread causes further losses of 10-30 per cent over the period 30-70 seconds. Losses of thiamine in various meat products using different cooking techniques are shown in Table 11. Natural constituents of blueberries and coffee destroy thiamine. Plant phenols degrade the vitamin

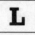 

under the influence of enzyme oxidases. Thiaminases, enzymes that destroy thiamine, are present in various fish and crustaceans but adequate cooking removes the enzymes and preserves the vitamin.

*Riboflavin* — is stable to oxygen, acid and heat up to 130°C. Unstable to alkalis and light. Readily lost by leaching from chopped foods in wet processing and cooking.

Light in presence of alkali converts riboflavin to lumiflavin which in turn destroys vitamin C. In milk 5 per cent lumiflavin can cause 50 per cent loss in vitamin C content. Milk exposed to light in summer loses 90 per cent of its riboflavin content in full sunshine in two hours; 45 per cent in cloudy weather and 30 per cent when sky is completely clouded over. Room lighting causes 30 per cent loss within 24 hours. Light affects riboflavin content of small bread rolls: supermarket lighting destroyed 17 per cent of the content in 24 hours; 13 per cent when rolls were wrapped in amber plastic film and 2 per cent when wrapped in orange plastic.

In the dark, under slightly acid conditions, riboflavin is completely stable, e.g. after 48 days in cold storage beef has the same vitamin content as that immediately after slaughter.

Milk loses riboflavin when heated. On boiling there are losses of 12-25 per cent; in pasteurization these losses are 14 per cent. Similar losses occur in meat cooking and in all cases losses are greater in the presence of light. Dry curing of meat gives rise to 40 per cent loss of riboflavin content; wet curing causes similar losses.

*Nicotinic acid* — is very stable and leaching causes the only losses. It is unaffected by heat, air, light, acidity and alkalinity, and by sulphite. One of the few vitamins to be liberated by cooking processes since in many cereals it is bound to starches and proteins in a complex called niacytin which is not digested in the gastro-intestinal tract. In wheat flour, 77 per cent of the nicotinic acid is in a bound form that is completely liberated by baking with alkaline baking powder. In Mexico corn is soaked overnight in lime water before making tortillas in order to free the vitamin.

Some loss of nicotinic acid when cooking meat but all can be recovered from the juices. Roasting beef and pork at 150°C loses less than 10 per cent of the vitamin; at temperatures of 205°C (which give an internal temperature of 98°C) losses are 30 per cent. Dry curing of meat gives rise to no losses of nicotinic acid; wet curing causes 20 per cent of it to be leached but this is recoverable.

No nicotinic acid is lost in the pasteurization and sterilization of milk or in the production of dried milk and dried egg.

*Pyridoxine* — is very stable to heat but pyridoxal and pyridoxamine are more sensitive. Stability in milk during sterilization or drying is reduced due to interaction with milk proteins. Losses can occur up to 20 per cent during milk sterilization; higher temperatures cause more serious losses. No destruction of pyridoxine during cooking. Three forms of the vitamin are all stable to air, acid and alkali. Canning of beans gives rise to 20 per cent loss into blanching water and 15 per cent in steam but all can be recovered by utilizing the water. Losses into thawed fluids of 20-40 per cent can occur when frozen vegetables are cooked.

*Folic acid* — unstable only in the free form. Losses are 10 per cent on steam blanching, 20 per cent in pressure cooking and 25-50 per cent in boiling vegetables. Can be destroyed by oxidation. Losses from sterilized milk can vary from 20-100 per cent depending on time of contact with air. If vitamin C is present, there is protective effect and no folic acid is lost. If vitamin C is destroyed by subsequent reheating, folic acid is also oxidized.

Is sensitive to sunlight and destruction is catalyzed by riboflavin. In one year, 30 per cent of folic acid was lost in tomato juice stored in clear glass bottles compared with only 7 per cent in those with dark glass.

Cumulative losses of folic acid occur in food processing. Soaking beans for twelve hours leaches out 5 per cent that is recoverable; blanching in water at 100°C causes a loss of 20 per cent in five minutes, 25 per cent in ten minutes and 45 per cent in 20 minutes, only some of which is recoverable; sterilization in the can at 118°C for 30 minutes destroys 10 per cent of that left. No further losses occur while in the can.

Baking bread destroys one-third of the folate present in the original flour. Vitamin is not affected by any of the improvers used in commercial baking. Losses from foods such as vegetables, fruits and dairy products average 70 per cent of the free folic acid and 45 per cent of the total free and conjugated varieties during overall processing and cooking.

*Vitamin B$_{12}$* — unstable in the presence of alkali but stable under all other conditions of cooking. Light may destroy some but proteins in the food appear to protect the vitamin. Leaching represents main loss in food preparation.

*Pantothenic acid* — stable under most cooking methods that are carried out in neutral conditions but destroyed by heat both on acid and alkaline side of neutrality. Wheat suffers a 60 per cent loss during manufacturing procedures involving baking powder. Meat losses are 30 per cent during cooking but most is recoverable as it is due to leaching. Six to eight per cent is lost from meats over periods up to twelve months in deep frozen state.

*Biotin* — nothing is known about its stability in cooking processes.

*Vitamin C* — most unstable of all the vitamins. Heating cabbage at 100°C (boiling point of water) for 20 minutes reduced vitamin C content by 70 per cent; simmering at 70-80°C for 60 minutes reduced it by 90 per cent. Some vitamin C can be recovered from cooking water (see Table 12). Pre-heating the cabbage virtually removes the rest of the vitamin.

Vitamin C is lost in food: by oxidation with ascorbic acid oxidase (an enzyme released by bruising or wilting); by air oxidation, catalysed by copper; and by leaching into processing and cooking water. Dehydro-ascorbic acid is produced by oxidation but this can revert to the vitamin and is active. Blanching or rapid heating of the raw food destroys the ascorbic acid oxidase and so preserves the vitamin. Vitamin C losses in vegetables during household cooking processes are shown in Table 12. Once air is excluded as in canned or bottled foods, vitamin C is very stable.

**Table 12: Vitamin C losses in vegetables during cooking**

|  | Percentage destroyed | Percentage extracted | Percentage retained |
|---|---|---|---|
| *Green vegetables* | | | |
| Boiling (long time, much water) | 10-15 | 45-60 | 22-45 |
| Boiling (short time, little water) | 10-15 | 15-30 | 55-75 |
| Steaming | 30-40 | <10 | 60-70 |
| Pressure cooking | 20-40 | <10 | 60-80 |
| *Root vegetables (unsliced)* | | | |
| Boiling | 10-20 | 15-25 | 55-75 |
| Steaming | 30-50 | <10 | 50-70 |
| Pressure cooking | 45-55 | <10 | 45-55 |

Fruits rich in anthocyanins (natural coloring pigments) lose vitamin C more rapidly, e.g. strawberries can lose 40-60 per cent in processing and four months' storage at blood heat (37°C); raspberries and black currants are even less stable. Vitamin C in apple juice is very unstable; 50 per cent loss in 4-8 days and 95 per cent loss in sixteen days when stored in refrigerator (5°C). Some stability is conferred by sulphur dioxide but this is lost once container is opened.

Orange drinks lose 30-50 per cent of their vitamin C content within eight days of opening bottle and as much as 90 per cent after 3-4 months, even at refrigerated temperatures. Percentage losses of vitamin C from fruit pulp exposed to air are shown in Table 13. Shaking the bottle after opening accelerates breakdown of vitamin C.

**Table 13: Percentage losses of vitamin C from fruit pulp**

|  | Exposure in days | | | |
|---|---|---|---|---|
|  | 8 | 15 | 35 | 40 |
| Stored full | 5 | — | 10 | — |
| Opened | 15 | 30 | — | 90 |
| Stored half full | 30 | 60 | 70 | 100 |

Available vitamin C from peas (as percentage of that in raw vegetables) at various stages of processing is given in Table 14.

**Table 14: Percentage of original vitamin C content in peas at various stages of processing**

|  | Blanching | Sterilizing | Freezing | Leached out | Thawing | As eaten |
|---|---|---|---|---|---|---|
| Fresh | — | — | — | 48 | — | 44 |
| Canned | 70 | 45 | — | 18 | — | 6 |
| Frozen | 75 | — | 56 | — | 41 | 17 |

The vitamin C content of potatoes in relation to age and cooking methods is shown in Table 15.

**Table 15: Vitamin C content of potatoes in relation to age and cooking methods**

|  | In mg per 100g | | |
|---|---|---|---|
|  | Raw | Boiled and peeled | Baked with skin |
| Main crop — |  |  |  |
| fresh, dry | 30 | 18 | 24 |
| Stored 1-3 months | 20 | 12 | 16 |
| Stored 4-5 months | 15 | 9 | 12 |
| Stored 6-7 months | 10 | 6 | 8 |
| Stored 8-9 months | 8 | 4.8 | 6.4 |

*Losses of vitamin C in storage* — vitamin C is lost steadily from potatoes once they leave the ground and are stored:

Main crop, freshly dug contain 30mg per 100g.
After 1-3 months' storage contain 20mg per 100g.
After 4-5 months' storage contain 15mg per 100g.
After 6-7 months' storage contain 10mg per 100g.
After 8-9 months' storage contain 8mg per 100g.

*Vitamin D* — regarded as being very stable but few studies carried out. It withstands smoking of fish, pasteurization and sterilization of milk and drying of eggs. Probably loses between 25 and 35 per cent of activity during the spray-drying of milk but this is allowed for in fortification.

*Vitamin E* — very sensitive to oxidation, particularly in the presence of heat and alkali. Serious degradation in frozen foods, e.g. potato chips lose 48 per cent of their vitamin E after two weeks at room temperature; 70 per cent after four weeks and 77 per cent in eight weeks. Even at deep-freeze temperatures (-12°C) vitamin E losses can total 68 per cent after two weeks. French-fried potatoes at the same low temperature can lose 68 per cent and 74 per cent of the vitamin after one month and two months respectively.

Processing and refining of cereals lead to wholesome losses of vitamin E. The most serious is the decrease in the vitamin content of white flour (92 per cent) when it is produced from whole-wheat grains. Whole-wheat bread provides 2.2mg per 100g compared with only 0.23mg in the white variety because the wheat germ is removed and bleaching agents destroy vitamin E.

Cooking food in fats destroys 70-90 per cent of the vitamin E content. Greatest losses happen in the presence of rancid fats and oils and these cannot always be detected by taste. Continual use of cooking fats and oils (e.g. in deep fryer) consistently destroys the vitamin in the food being fried.

Tocopherol esters are more stable than the free tocopherol. Only 10-20 per cent of the ester was destroyed under conditions that completely inactivated the free vitamin.

Boiling destroys 30 per cent of the vitamin E in sprouts, cabbages and carrots. Canning of vegetables leads to even greater losses, up to 80 per cent of the original content.

---

**low-fat margarine,** fortified with vitamins A and D to contain (in µg per 100g): vitamin A 900; vitamin D 7.94; vitamin E 4mg per 100g. Completely devoid of all water-soluble vitamins. *See also* margarine.

---

**lumbago,** pain, tenderness and stiffness in the back muscles. Has been relieved by high doses (up to 600mg) of thiamine. May also respond to 2g calcium pantothenate daily.

---

**lung cancer,** *see* cancer.

---

**lychees,** canned variety contain reduced levels of B vitamins compared with raw fruit but vitamin C is drastically decreased. Traces only of carotene and vitamin E. B vitamins present are (in mg per 100g), for the raw fruit and canned variety respectively: thiamine 0.04, 0.03; riboflavin 0.04, 0.03; nicotinic acid 0.4, 0.3. Vitamin C level of raw fruit is 40mg per 100g, but that of canned fruit is only 8mg per 100g.

---

# M

---

**macaroni,** pasta prepared from wheat flour. Trace only of vitamin E in the raw and boiled pasta. Completely devoid of carotene and vitamin C. Reduced concentrations of B vitamins in boiling because of water uptake. B vitamins present are (in mg per 100g), for the raw and boiled pasta respectively: thiamine 0.14, 0.01; riboflavin 0.06, 0.01; nicotinic acid 4.8, 1.2; pyridoxine 0.06, 0.01; pantothenic acid 0.3, trace. Folic acid levels are (in µg per 100g), for raw and boiled macaroni respectively 11 and 2; biotin levels are 1 and trace.

---

**McCollum, Elmer V.,** Canadian biochemist who demonstrated presence of vitamin A in some fatty foods culminating in its isolation in 1926.

---

**mandarin oranges,** *canned* variety are a useful source of vitamin C, providing also some B vitamins and carotene. Carotene content is 50µg per 100g; trace only of vitamin E. B vitamins present are (in mg per 100g):

thiamine 0.07; riboflavin 0.02; nicotinic acid 0.3; pyridoxine 0.03; pantothenic acid 0.15. Folic acid is 8µg per 100g; that of biotin is 0.8µg per 100g. Vitamin C content is 14mg per 100g.

---

**mangoes,**    rich source of carotene. In the ripe, orange-colored mangoes, both raw and canned, there are 1.2mg carotene per 100g. Carotene content varies according to the color and unripe, green fruit contain about 120µg carotene per 100g. Vitamin E is not detectable. B vitamins present are (in mg per 100g), for raw and canned mangoes respectively: thiamine 0.03, 0.02; riboflavin 0.04, 0.03; nicotinic acid 0.2, 0.2; pantothenic acid 0.16, 0.15. Folic acid and biotin have not been detected. Good source of vitamin C at levels of 30mg (range 10-180mg) per 100g in the raw state and 10mg per 100g in the canned variety.

---

**margarine,**    both hard and soft are fortified with vitamins A and D to contain (in µg per 100g): vitamin A 900; vitamin D 7.94. Good source of vitamin E, providing 8.0mg per 100g. Traces only of all B vitamins but contains no vitamin C. *See also* low-fat margarine.

---

**marmalade,**    provides useful sources of carotene and vitamin C but only traces of other vitamins. Carotene content is 50µg per 100g with traces only of vitamin E. B vitamins present are traces of thiamine, riboflavin, nicotinic acid, pyridoxine, pantothenic acid and biotin. Folic acid level is 5µg per 100g. Vitamin C content is 10mg per 100g.

---

**marzipan,**    vitamins are provided by almonds, lemon juice and eggs. Vitamin A content is 10µg per 100g, but carotene is absent. Vitamin D content of 0.13µg per 100g. Good provider of vitamin E at 9.1mg per 100g. B vitamins present are (in mg per 100g): thiamine 0.12; riboflavin 0.45; nicotinic acid 2.4; pyridoxine 0.06; pantothenic acid 0.35. Folic acid level is 45µg per 100g; biotin level is 2µg per 100g. Vitamin C content is 2mg per 100g.

---

**meats,**    cooking losses. Average losses in meats and poultry during various cooking methods are shown in Table 16. Liver and other organ meats are the only significant sources of vitamin C and losses average 20 per cent in all cooking methods.

**Table 16: Average percentage losses of vitamins in meats and poultry during cooking**

|  | Roasting, frying, broiling | Stewing, boiling |
|---|---|---|
| Vitamin A | 0 | 0 |
| Vitamin E | 20 | 20 |
| Vitamin $B_{12}$ | 20 | 20 |
| Biotin | 10 | 10 |
| Thiamine | 20 | 60 |
| Riboflavin | 20 | 30 |
| Nicotinic acid | 20 | 50 |
| Pyridoxine | 20 | 50 |
| Pantothenic acid | 20 | 40 |
| Folic acid | 10 | 30 |

**megaloblastic anemia,** characterized by appearance of large, immature red blood cells with shortened life-span. May be due to deficiency of folic acid, vitamin $B_{12}$ or pyridoxine. Only treatment is to replace specific deficient vitamin.

**megavitamin therapy,** treating certain conditions with doses of vitamins far above the levels found even in good diets. Using vitamins as medicines but without the side-effects noted with drugs. Has been used successfully in treating arthritis, autism, colds, heart disease, hyperactivity, learning disabilities, respiratory infections, schizophrenia, senile dementia. *See* individual complaint for treatment.

**Mellanby, E.,** British doctor who demonstrated that rickets is a nutritional disease that responds to a factor present in cod-liver oil, later named vitamin D.

**melons,** *Cantaloupe,* raw, edible portion is very rich source of carotene, providing also a good amount of vitamin C. The orange-colored flesh contains 2.0mg carotene per 100g plus 0.1mg per 100g of vitamin E. B vitamins present are (in mg per 100g): thiamine 0.05; riboflavin 0.03; nicotinic acid 0.5; pyridoxine 0.07; pantothenic acid 0.23. Folic acid level is 30µg per 100g; biotin has not been detected. Vitamin C content is 25mg per 100g.

*Honeydew,* raw, edible portion is moderate source of carotene but provides good amounts of vitamin C. Carotene content is 100µg per 100g for the green-colored flesh; vitamin E level is 0.1mg per 100g. B vitamins present are (in mg per 100g): thiamine 0.05; riboflavin 0.03; nicotinic acid 0.5; pyridoxine 0.07; pantothenic acid 0.23. Folic acid level is 30µg per 100g; biotin is absent. Vitamin C content is 25mg per 100g.

*Watermelon,* raw, edible portion is poor source of all vitamins except pantothenic acid and C. Carotene is 20µg per 100g; vitamin E level is 0.1mg per 100g. B vitamins present are (in mg per 100g): thiamine 0.02; riboflavin 0.02; nicotinic acid 0.3; pyridoxine 0.07; pantothenic acid 1.55. Provides small amount of folic acid (3µg per 100g) but no biotin. Vitamin C content is 5mg per 100g.

---

**memory,**    when faulty may be symptom of thiamine deficiency. Treat with adequate doses (up to 50mg daily) of vitamin $B_1$. When associated with age may respond to choline. *See* senile dementia. Claims that RNA intake may help improve memory, particularly in the aged.

---

**menaphthone,**    *see* $K_3$ vitamin.

---

**menaquinone,**    *see* $K_2$ vitamin.

---

**Meniere's disease,**    a disorder characterized by recurrent severe vertigo, deafness, tinnitus (noises in the ear), nausea and vomiting. Some relief gained by following regime: thiamine (10-25mg); riboflavin (10-25mg); 50:50 mixture of nicotinic acid:nicotinamide (100-250mg); all four times daily for two weeks. If relief obtained, reduce all vitamins to dose that maintains relief and continue.

---

**menopause,**    period in a woman's life when her secretion of female sex hormones slows down and eventually ceases. Characterized by hot flushes, headaches, giddiness, nervousness, depression, excessive menstrual flow, increase in weight, pruritus (itching) in sexual parts.

Vitamin E (100IU with each meal) claimed to relieve hot flushes, headaches, nervousness. Pyridoxine (50-100mg daily) may help relieve depression. Iron (15mg) and vitamin C (200mg) daily will help replace blood losses. Calcium (200mg) and vitamin D (6.25μg) will help prevent calcium loss from bones induced by deficiency of estrogens.

---

**menstruation,**   monthly breakdown of lining of uterus leading to loss of blood in the menstrual flow.

Blood loss replaced by adequate intakes of mineral iron (24mg) with vitamin C (100mg); vitamin E (100IU); folic acid (25μg) and vitamin $B_{12}$ (5μg). Mild depression that occurs just before menstruation often responds to pyridoxine — *see* depression. Irregular or painful menstrual periods may respond to bioflavonoids (1000mg daily).

---

**mental ability,**   may be increased in normal children with thiamine (10mg), vitamin C (100mg) and vitamin E (100IU) daily to ensure adequate intakes and so maximum potential.

---

**mental disturbance,**   can be related to mild deficiencies of vitamins, particularly thiamine, riboflavin, nicotinamide, pyridoxine, folic acid, vitamin $B_{12}$. Individual may also be vitamin-dependent, requiring larger intakes than can be obtained from diet. *See* autism, depression, megavitamin therapy, schizophrenia, senile dementia.

---

**Mervyn, Leonard,**   British biochemist who discovered ubiquinone (coenzyme Q), a fat-soluble, vitamin-like substance, in man. Ubiquinone plays an important part in cell respiration, particularly in the heart.

First to synthesize vitamin $B_{12}$ coenzymes, which enabled him to demonstrate relationship between vitamin $B_{12}$ and folic acid in megaloblastic anemia. Studied vitamin changes in disease states and the effect of medicinal drugs on nutritional status.

---

**meso-inositol,**   *see* inositol.

---

**metformin,**   anti-diabetic drug. Prevents absorption of vitamin $B_{12}$.

---

**methotrexate,**   anti-cancer drug. Immuno-suppressant. Impairs folic acid utilization.

**migraine,**   a particular type of headache caused by constriction of the blood-vessels followed by their dilation which gives rise to pulsating pain. Characterized by nausea, vomiting and visual disturbances in severe cases.

Vitamin therapy includes whole vitamin B complex (10mg potency) three times daily plus nicotinamide (100mg), calcium pantothenate (100mg), pyridoxine (50mg) all three times daily. If regime prevents attacks, reduce gradually to that intake that maintains relief.

**milk,**   good source of all the vitamins but seasonal variation with regard to fat-soluble vitamins.

*Whole cow's milk in summer* contains (in mg per 100g): vitamin A 0.035; carotene 0.022; thiamine 0.04; riboflavin 0.19; nicotinic acid 0.86; pyridoxine 0.04; folic acid 0.005; pantothenic acid 0.35; biotin 0.002; vitamin E 0.1; vitamin C 1.5; vitamin $B_{12}$ 0.3μg; vitamin D 0.03μg. *In winter,* fat-soluble vitamins only reduced to (per 100g): vitamin A 26μg; carotene 13μg; vitamin D 0.013μg; vitamin E 0.07mg.

*Sterilized summer milk* contains (per 100g): vitamin A 31μg; carotene 18μg; vitamin D 0.022μg; thiamine 0.03mg; riboflavin 0.19mg; nicotinic acid 0.86mg; pyridoxine 0.03mg; folic acid 0.004mg; pantothenic acid 0.35mg; biotin 0.002mg; vitamin $B_{12}$ 0.2μg; vitamin C 0.8mg; vitamin E 0.09mg.

*Skimmed milk* is essentially devoid of fat-soluble vitamins but water-soluble B vitamins and C are contained in same concentration as in whole milk. *Dried skimmed milk* is rich source of B vitamins and C, providing (in mg per 100g): thiamine 0.42; riboflavin 1.6; nicotinic acid 9.75; pyridoxine 0.25; folic acid 0.021; pantothenic acid 3.5; biotin 0.016; vitamin C 6.0; vitamin $B_{12}$ 3.0μg.

*Goat's milk* contains all vitamins in similar concentrations to those in cow's milk.

*Human milk* shows some variation to cow's milk, providing (in mg per 100g): vitamin A 0.6; thiamine 0.02; riboflavin 0.03; nicotinic acid 0.69; pyridoxine 0.01; folic acid 0.005; pantothenic acid 0.25; vitamin C 3.7; vitamin E 0.34; vitamin D 0.025μg; biotin 0.7μg.

The percentage losses of vitamins in the processing of milk are shown in Table 17. Other vitamins are unaffected during processing.

**Table 17: Percentage losses of vitamins in processing milk**

| | Thiamine | Riboflavin | Pyridoxine | Vit. $B_{12}$ | Folic acid | Vit. C | Vit. E |
|---|---|---|---|---|---|---|---|
| Pasteurization | 10 | 0 | 0 | 0 | 5 | 25 | 0 |
| Sterilization | 20 | 0 | 20 | 20 | 30 | 60 | 0 |
| UHT | 10 | 0 | 10 | 5 | 20 | 30 | 0 |
| UHT (after 3 months) | 10 | 0 | 35 | 20 | 50 | 100 | 0 |
| Boiled, pasteurized | 0 | 10 | 10 | 5 | 20 | 50 | 20 |

**mincemeat,** dried fruit and nuts provide most of the vitamins present. Carotene content is 10µg per 100g. B vitamins present are (in mg per 100g): thiamine 0.03; riboflavin 0.02; nicotinic acid 0.3; pyridoxine 0.10; pantothenic acid 0.03. Traces only of folic acid, biotin and vitamin C.

**molasses,** contains the following B vitamins in mg per 100g: thiamine 0.03; riboflavin 0.05; nicotinic acid 10.0; pyridoxine 0.10; pantothenic acid 1.2. Contains also choline (16.0mg per 100g); inositol (120mg per 100g). Black variety contains traces only of thiamine, riboflavin, nicotinic acid, pyridoxine, folic acid and biotin.

**Moore, T.,** British biochemist, leading researcher in vitamin A, who proved unequivocally that carotene is a precursor of the vitamin.

**morning sickness,** *see* nausea.

**Morton, R. A.,** British scientist at Liverpool University who first worked out the mechanism of vitamin A in the process of sight.

**mucous membranes,** wet surfaces of the body including nose, eyes, mouth, respiratory system, digestive tract, anus and genital tracts.
Vitamin A protects all mucous membranes and maintains their health. Deficiency of vitamin leads to drying out of membranes resulting in ulceration and liability to infection — *see* keratinization.

Inflammation can result from deficiency of nicotinic acid and riboflavin. Polluted atmosphere can destroy membrane — best protected with vitamins A and E. Tobacco smoking irritates mucous membranes of respiratory tract — best protected with beta-carotene.

**mulberries,**  in the raw state provide good quantity of vitamin C but only small quantities of B vitamins. Traces only of carotene and vitamin E. B vitamins present are (in mg per 100g): thiamine 0.05; riboflavin 0.04; nicotinic acid 0.6; pyridoxine 0.05; pantothenic acid 0.25. Biotin level is 0.4µg per 100g but no folic acid has been detected. Vitamin C content is 10mg per 100g.

**mung beans,**  when raw supply only carotene at level of 24µg per 100g. B vitamins present in good quantities are (in mg per 100g): thiamine 0.45; riboflavin 0.20; nicotinic acid 5.5; pyridoxine 0.50; pantothenic acid absent. Good source of folic acid at 140µg per 100g. Negligible vitamin C present.

**muscle pain,**  may be related to biotin deficiency. Treat with 2 to 5mg daily by mouth.

**muscle spasms,**  also known as restless legs. Often occurs during sleep and relieved by walking or moving affected leg. Treated with vitamin E (100IU with each meal *or* 400IU in one dose daily).

**muscles,**  need good blood supply and efficient conversion of nutrients into energy for maximum performance. Vitamin E (400IU daily) essential to maintain healthy blood-vessels. Vitamin C (500mg daily) essential for production of carnitine, needed for muscle energy. *See* carnitine.

**muscular dystrophy,**  muscle disease characterized by progressive weakness and degeneration of muscle fibers but without evidence of nerve degeneration. Symptom of vitamin E deficiency in many animal species and can be cured by vitamin treatment. No evidence of relationship between vitamin E and human muscular dystrophy but occasionally cases have responded to high doses of vitamin E, preferably with the trace mineral selenium.

Benefit in rare cases claimed with ubiquinone, a natural vitamin-like substance, produced in the body under the influence of vitamin E.

---

**mushrooms,**    completely devoid of carotene with traces only of vitamin E. Some reduction of B vitamins content when fried; concentrations (in mg per 100g) are, for raw and fried respectively: thiamine 0.10, 0.07; riboflavin 0.40, 0.35; nicotinic acid 4.6, 4.4; pyridoxine 0.10, 0.06; pantothenic acid 2.0, 1.4. Folic acid content little reduced, from 23 to 20$\mu$g per 100g on frying. Small amount of vitamin C present, 3.0 and 1.0mg per 100g for raw and fried mushrooms respectively.

---

**myelin,**    fatty sheath that covers nerves and spinal cord and acts as insulator. Composed of cholesterol, PUFA and phosphatidyl choline complexed with lipid called sphingosine. Myelin loss due to degeneration is factor in multiple sclerosis. Vitamin $B_{12}$ and PUFA essential for healthy myelin sheath.

---

**myocardial infarction,**    *see* heart disease.

---

**myo-inositol,**    *see* inositol.

---

# N

---

**natural vitamins,**    those that are:

1.   derived from natural sources (e.g., d-alpha tocopherol);
2.   produced by fermentation (e.g., vitamin $B_{12}$);
3.   presented in a natural environment (e.g., vitamin E in wheat germ oil or soybean oil);
4.   presented in a food (e.g., vitamin B complex in yeast).

*Advantages* are:

1.  biologically more active (e.g., d-alpha tocopherol);
2.  better absorbed (e.g., fat-soluble vitamins need fats or oils present as well);
3.  better utilized in presence of other factors (e.g., vitamin C and bioflavonoids occur in foods together and function in body together);
4.  retained by body longer (e.g., natural vitamin E).

---

**nausea,**  feeling of discomfort in region of stomach with aversion to food and tendency to vomit. Side-effect of many medicinal drugs.

*Morning sickness* — nausea of the early stages of pregnancy. Has been treated with pyridoxine (25mg with each meal).

*Travel sickness* — nausea associated with various forms of travel. Has been treated with pyridoxine (25mg) and ginger (160mg) before trip and if necessary during it. Half dose effective for children.

---

**nectarines,**  raw, edible portion provides useful quantities of carotene and vitamin C. Carotene content is $500\mu g$ per 100g; vitamin E has not been detected. B vitamins present are (in mg per 100g): thiamine 0.02; riboflavin 0.05; nicotinic acid 1.0; pyridoxine 0.02; pantothenic acid 0.15. Folic acid level is $5\mu g$ per 100g. Vitamin C content is 8mg per 100g.

---

**neomycin,**  antibiotic. Prevents absorption of vitamin D.

---

**nervous system,**  health depends upon adequate vitamin B complex and vitamin E. Thiamine at intakes between 50 and 600mg daily has relieved sciatica, trigeminal neuralgia, facial paralysis, optic neuritis and peripheral neuritis. Psychosis and mental deterioration have responded to vitamin $B_{12}$, preferably by injection.

Choline is of benefit in some cases of Alzheimer's disease and senile dementia. A combination of vitamin E and inositol has helped in some nerve diseases associated with muscle degeneration. Huntington's chorea treated with high potencies of whole vitamin B complex has relieved mental deterioration of the disease. Mild depression will often respond to vitamin $B_6$ therapy alone.

Nicotinic acid in high doses (1-3g daily) has been used successfully in schizophrenia. Paraesthesia relieved by 50mg pyridoxine daily.

Deficiencies of thiamine, riboflavin, nicotinamide, pyridoxine and vitamin $B_{12}$ all cause damage to nervous system. Preferable therefore to treat any mild mental or nervous condition with high potency of whole vitamin B complex.

---

**neuritis,** general term for degeneration and inflammation of one or more nerves. Symptom rather than disease.

*Optic,* inflammation of the eye nerve.

*Peripheral,* affecting simultaneously several nerves, usually those of the limbs. Caused by thiamine deficiency, diabetes, alcohol, heavy metal poisoning. Also known as polyneuritis.

Treatment — *see* nervous system.

---

**new potatoes,** when boiled lose some B vitamins but mainly vitamin C. Canning potatoes causes further losses of B vitamins but not vitamin C. Concentrations of B vitamins (in mg per 100g), for boiled new and canned new potatoes respectively, are: thiamine 0.11, 0.02; riboflavin 0.03, 0.03; nicotinic acid 1.6, 1.0; pyridoxine 0.20, 0.16; pantothenic acid 0.20, 0.10. Folic acid stable at concentrations of 10 and 11µg per 100g respectively. Vitamin C levels are 18 and 17mg per 100g respectively. *See also* potatoes.

---

**niacin,** water-soluble vitamin, member of the vitamin B complex. Synonymous with nicotinic acid. Presented also as nicotinamide (synonymous with niacinamide), the active form in the body, in supplements. Known as vitamin $B_3$ (USA) and vitamin $B_5$ (Europe) in the past. Now generally accepted as vitamin $B_3$. Also known as vitamin PP (pellagra-preventing) or PP Factor. Nicotinic acid known since 1867 but demonstrated as a vitamin only in 1937 by Dr. Conrad Elvehjem.

*Richest sources* (in mg per 100g) are: yeast extract (67); dried brewer's yeast (37.9); wheat bran (32.6); nuts (21.3); pig liver (19.4); chicken (11.6); soy flour (10.6); meat (9.5 to 10.4); fatty fish (10.4); wheat grains (8.1); cheese (6.2); dried fruits (5.6); whole-wheat bread (5.6); white fish (4.9); brown rice (4.7); wheat germ (4.2); oatflakes (4.1); eggs (3.7); legumes (3.4).

*Produced* in body from amino acid tryptophane, 60mg giving rise to 1mg nicotinic acid. Above figures include that contributed by tryptophane.

*Very stable* during cooking processes. Lost only by leaching into water and in drips from thawing frozen foods.

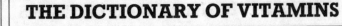

*Functions* as respiratory coenzymes nicotinamide adenine dinucleotide (NAD) and nicotinamide adenine dinucleotide phosphate (NADP) in tissue oxidations. Assist in production of energy from carbohydrates, fats and protein. Essential for proper utilization of brain and nerves and for maintaining healthy skin, tongue and digestive organs.

*Deficiency* causes disease called pellagra (in dogs canine black tongue).

*Deficiency symptoms* of pellagra are the three D's, dermatitis, diarrhea and dementia leading to fourth, death. Early symptoms are muscular weakness, general fatigue, loss of appetite, indigestion and minor skin complaints. Also insomnia, irritability, stress and depression associated with nervous system. Gastro-intestinal symptoms are nausea, vomiting, inflamed mouth and digestive tract. Skin lesions include rashes, dry, scaly skin, wrinkles and coarse texture.

*Deficiency in animals* affects mainly the skin and digestive organs. Symptoms are loss of appetite, retarded growth, weakness, digestive disorders and diarrhea; digestive tract is inflamed with ulcers and bleeding in the large intestine; coat is rough with scaly dermatitis; anemia. In dog dark blue pigmentation of tongue with disturbed reflexes, paralysis and epilepsy.

*Recommended daily intakes* in the USA are 9.0mg for children under 4 years and 20mg for all others, including pregnant and lactating women. In the UK, levels range from 5mg (less than 1 year) to 19mg (17 years) in both males and females; 18mg (adult men) and 15mg (adult women) increasing to 18mg (during pregnancy) and 21mg (during lactation). WHO levels similar.

*Increased intakes* required by alcohol drinkers and those taking anti-leukemia drugs based on 6-mercaptopurine. 50mg extra is sufficient.

*Toxicity* of nicotinamide is low but large doses (greater than 3g daily) may cause depression and liver malfunction. Avoid high doses during first 56 days of pregnancy. Nicotinic acid more toxic. Symptoms include flushing of face, sensation of heat and pounding headache. Sometimes dry skin, itching and boils. Abdominal cramps, diarrhea and nausea. Occasionally mild gout symptoms. Avoid high doses of nicotinic acid when suffering from gastric or duodenal ulcers.

No official limit on potency in supplements.

*Therapy* with high doses of nicotinamide or nicotinic acid in schizophrenia, particularly in children. Both used to wean alcoholics off alcohol, tobacco smokers off smoking. Both used to treat symptoms of arthritis. Nicotinic acid alone specifically lowers blood cholesterol and blood fats.

**niacinamide,**  active form of nicotinic acid. Known also as nicotinamide.

---

**nicotinamide,**  active metabolic form of nicotinic acid.

---

**nicotinic acid,**  niacin, vitamin $B_3$.

---

**night blindness,**  inability to see in the dark due solely to vitamin A deficiency.

---

**nitrates,**  *see* nitrosamines.

---

**nitrites,**  *see* nitrosamines.

---

**nitritocobalamin,**  *see* $B_{12}$ vitamin.

---

**nitrofurantoin,**  urinary anti-infective. Impairs folic acid utilization.

---

**nitrosamines,**  toxic substances associated with certain types of cancer. Readily formed in the digestive tract from amines and nitrites, both present in food, drugs, cosmetics and the environment. Nitrites used extensively as food preservatives and readily formed from nitrates. Nitrosamines more likely to be produced in stomach in absence of acid.

Vitamin C prevents formation of nitrosamines and neutralizes preformed variety, so vitamin should be taken at every meal.

---

**nucleic acids,**  comprise both ribonucleic acids (RNA) and de-oxyribonucleic acids (DNA). Essential components of all living cells, they are necessary for cell growth and hereditary information. Reduced synthesis leads to consequences of ageing including poor memory. Have been used to slow down ageing process, usually given by injection.

Vitamins needed for healthy RNA and DNA production in human beings include vitamin A, vitamin E, pyridoxine, folic acid, vitamin $B_{12}$ and choline.

Present in dried yeast to extent of 12 per cent of weight.

---

**nuts,**　kernels of all nuts are completely devoid of carotene and in the ripe state contain traces only of vitamin C. Provide good quantities of vitamin E but only two types present, alpha-tocopherol and gamma-tocopherol. Brazil nuts, chestnuts, peanuts and walnut kernels contain mainly gamma-tocopherol. Individual figures for all kernels are total tocopherols. All kernels supply good quantities of the B vitamins. *See* individual nuts.

# O

---

**oatmeal,**　when raw is rich source of B vitamins providing (in mg per 100g): thiamine 0.50; riboflavin 0.10; nicotinic acid 3.8; pyridoxine 0.12; folic acid 0.060; pantothenic acid 1.0; biotin 0.020; vitamin E 0.9. Devoid of vitamins A, D, C and carotene.

---

**oil of evening primrose,**　seed oil unique in containing substantial amounts of essential fatty acid (vitamin F) gammalinolenic acid (GLA). Usually produced in body from linoleic acid but claims that in some conditions synthesis blocked or not sufficient. Reports that GLA beneficial in: multiple sclerosis; in premenstrual syndrome; in skin disorders; in alcoholism; in hyperactivity in children; in arthritis and other inflammatory conditions; in disorders of the immune system. GLA functions as precursor of hormones known as prostaglandins. Usual intakes are 3 to 6 capsules per day (500mg oil containing 40mg GLA).

---

**okra,**　African plant known also as gumbo. Provides 90μg carotene per 100g in raw state. B vitamins present are (in mg per 100g): thiamine 0.10; riboflavin 0.10; nicotinic acid 1.3; pyridoxine 0.08; pantothenic acid 0.26. Good source of folic acid at 100μg per 100g. Good source of vitamin C at 25mg per 100g.

---

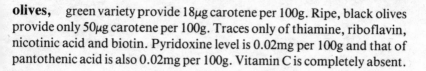

**olives,**   green variety provide 18μg carotene per 100g. Ripe, black olives provide only 50μg carotene per 100g. Traces only of thiamine, riboflavin, nicotinic acid and biotin. Pyridoxine level is 0.02mg per 100g and that of pantothenic acid is also 0.02mg per 100g. Vitamin C is completely absent.

---

**onions,**   contain no carotene and traces only of vitamin E. Poor source of B vitamins made poorer by boiling. Levels are (in mg per 100g), for raw and boiled respectively: thiamine 0.03, 0.02; riboflavin 0.05, 0.04; nicotinic acid 0.4, 0.2; pyridoxine 0.10, 0.06; pantothenic acid 0.14, 0.10. Folic acid levels (in μg per 100g) are 16, 8; and biotin levels are 0.9, 0.6 for raw and boiled onions respectively. Vitamin C content reduced from 10mg to 6mg per 100g on boiling. Frying virtually destroys the B vitamins and vitamin C; only 0.4mg nicotinic acid per 100g survives. *See also* scallions.

---

**orange drink,**   in undiluted form provides only traces of carotene, vitamin E, thiamine, riboflavin, nicotinic acid, pyridoxine, pantothenic acid, folic acid and biotin. Traces only of vitamin C but content may be increased to 20-60mg per 100g when fortified with the vitamin.

---

**orange juice,**   both sweetened and unsweetened canned varieties, provides similar concentrations of carotene, vitamin E and B vitamins with slightly higher levels of vitamin C in the unsweetened juice. Carotene content is 50μg per 100g; traces only of vitamin E. B vitamins present are (in mg per 100g): thiamine 0.07; riboflavin 0.02; nicotinic acid 0.3; pyridoxine 0.04; pantothenic acid 0.15. Folic acid level is 7μg per 100g; that of biotin is 1μg per 100g. Vitamin C content of sweetened and unsweetened canned juice is respectively 31 and 35mg per 100g.

---

**oranges,**   raw, edible portion has slightly higher levels of some of the water-soluble vitamins than the freshly expressed juice. Carotene contents (in μg per 100g) of both the raw, edible portion and fresh juice is 50μg per 100g; vitamin E level is 0.2mg per 100g in raw, edible portion but traces only in fresh juice. B vitamins present are (in μg per 100g), for raw, edible portion and fresh juice respectively: thiamine 0.10, 0.08; riboflavin 0.03, 0.02; nicotinic acid 0.3, 0.3; pyridoxine 0.06, 0.04; pantothenic acid 1.0, 0.8. Useful source of folic acid at 37μg per 100g in fruit and juice; biotin level is 1.0 and 0.8µg per 100g respectively. Vitamin C content at 50mg (range 40-60mg) per 100ml is identical in both fruit and juice.

*Reconstituted frozen juice* has same vitamin content as freshly expressed juice.

---

**organ meats,** supply vitamin C in addition to all other vitamins, unlike other meat products. Liver and kidney are particularly rich in vitamin A, nicotinic acid, pantothenic acid and vitamin $B_{12}$. *See* under individual foods.

---

**orotic acid,** known also as whey factor, animal galactose factor, vitamin $B_{13}$. No longer regarded as a vitamin.

*Richest food sources* are liquid whey and root vegetables but traces usually present in all foods containing the vitamin B complex.

*Stable* to food processing methods.

*Functions* as intermediate in metabolism of RNA and DNA in human beings and is produced in adequate quantities under normal circumstances.

Essential growth factor for micro-organisms.

*Deficiency in man* has not been reported.

*Deficiency in animals* has not been reported.

*Recommended dietary intakes* not set because need in diet not established.

*Toxicity* is low. Up to 4 grams orotic acid daily by mouth has caused no harm over many days treatment.

*Therapy* with orotic acid claimed in: multiple sclerosis (given by injection); in chronic hepatitis (given as calcium orotate over many months); in gout (4 grams daily of orotic acid for six days).

---

**orthomolecular medicine,** *see* megavitamin therapy.

---

**Osmond, Humphrey,** Canadian doctor who introduced megavitamin therapy in treatment of schizophrenia.

---

**osteomalacia,** a disease characterized by softening of the bones and low body levels of calcium due specifically to vitamin D deficiency in the adult. *See* vitamin D.

---

**osteoporosis,**   honeycombing of the bones due to loss of calcium that is not replaced. Associated mainly with post-menopausal period of life; long-term corticosteroid treatment. Symptoms are bone pain and ease of fracture. Treated with high intakes of calcium (1000mg daily) plus fluoride plus adequate vitamin D to ensure absorption (400IU) *or* hormone replacement therapy in post-menopausal state.

---

**otosclerosis,**   *see* deafness.

---

**oxygen,**   occasionally causes eye problems (retrolental fibroplasia) in premature babies in oxygen tents. Prevented by administration of vitamin E, usually by injection.

---

# P

---

**PABA,**   *see* para-aminobenzoic acid.

---

**pangamic acid,**   from "pan" everywhere and "gami" family. Water-soluble factor present in vitamin B complex. Also known as: $B_{15}$; vitamin $B_{15}$ (incorrectly); D-gluconic acid 6-(bis(1-methyl ethyl) amino acetate. First isolated from apricot pits in 1951 by father and son team of Drs. E. T. Krebs and E. T. Krebs, Jr. Present in supplements as calcium pangamate, sodium pangamate.

*Richest food sources* (in μg per 100g) are: rice bran (200); corn (150); dried brewer's yeast (128); oatflakes (106); wheat germ (70); apricot pits (65); wheat bran (31); pig liver (22); barley (12); whole-wheat flour (8).

*Unstable* to food processing. Lost and destroyed during cooking methods.

*Doubt* of correct structure of pangamic acid — now generally accepted as D-gluconic acid 6-(bis(1-methyl ethyl) amino acetate.

*Functions* as: stimulator of carriage of oxygen to blood from lungs and from blood to muscles and vital organs; as lipotropic agent to keep fat in solution; as detoxifying agent on poisons and free radicals; as stimulator of anti-stress hormone production.

*Deficiency in man* has not been reported. Symptoms are not specific but may be related to above functions.

*Deficiency in animals* has not been reported.

*Recommended dietary intakes* not set by any authority.

*Toxicity* is low. Safe in doses up to 300mg daily but occasional transient flushing of skin. Calcium pangamate better tolerated than sodium pangamate.

*Therapy* with pangamic acid claimed to be beneficial in heart disease, in atherosclerosis, in bronchial asthma, in diabetes.

---

**pantothenic acid,** from "panthos" meaning everywhere. Water-soluble vitamin, member of the vitamin B complex. Usually presented in supplements as calcium pantothenate, in cosmetics and toiletries as dexpanthenol and pantothenol. Known as vitamin $B_5$ (USA) and as vitamin $B_3$ (Europe) in the past. Now generally accepted as vitamin $B_5$. Originally referred to as chick antidermatitis factor. Anti-stress vitamin. Isolated from rice husks by Dr. R. J. Williams of the University of Texas in 1939. Natural form is D-pantothenic acid.

*Richest sources* (in mg per 100g) are: dried brewer's yeast (9.5); pig liver (6.5); yeast extract (3.8); pig kidney (3.0); fresh nuts (2.7); wheat bran (2.4); wheat germ (2.2); roasted nuts (2.1); soy flour (1.8); eggs (1.8); meats (0.7 to 1.1); poultry (1.2); oatflakes (0.9); legumes (0.75); dried fruits (0.70); corn (0.6); unpolished brown rice (0.6); whole-wheat bread (0.6); cheese (0.4); yoghurt (0.4); fruits, green-leaf vegetables and root vegetables (0.21 to 0.30). Substantial amounts produced by intestinal bacteria.

*Stable* in neutral solution, destroyed by heat in presence of acid (vinegar) and alkali (bicarbonate). Destroyed by dry-processing of foods; 50 per cent destruction and loss in refining flour; lost by leaching into cooking water and during deep freezing and thawing. Destroyed during roasting of meat.

*Functions* as constituent of coenzyme A needed for: production of energy; for converting cholesterol into anti-stress hormones; for control of fat metabolism; for antibody formation; for a healthy nervous system (converts choline to brain substance acetycholine); for detoxification of drugs.

*Deficiency* does not cause any specific diseases apart from "burning feet syndrome." Symptoms are aching, burning and throbbing in the feet. As they become more intense they develop into sharp, stabbing, shooting pains that spread to the knee causing agonizing pain.

*Deficiency symptoms* as described above but less specific are loss of appetite, indigestion, abdominal pain, respiratory infections, neuritis, arm and leg cramps, tenderness in the heel. Mental symptoms include insomnia, fatigue, depression and psychosis. Headaches, fast heart beat and low blood pressure have been noted.

*Deficiency in animals* gives rise to: graying of hair followed by alopecia; nerve degeneration with convulsions; dermatitis; intestinal distension and ulceration; fatty liver; degeneration of the adrenal glands; anemia with lack of production of white blood cells.

*Recommended dietary intakes* have not been set in the UK, WHO or USA but are thought to be a minimum of 10mg daily.

*Increased intakes* needed: during stress situations; after physical injury; after antibiotic therapy; while on streptomycin, neomycin, kanamycin and viomycin to lessen side-effects and toxicity; to increase resistance to infection; to reduce allergy effects on respiratory system, skin and gastro-intestinal tract.

*Toxicity* symptoms have not been reported for calcium pantothenate. Many grams have been taken without ill-effects.

*Therapy* with high doses of calcium pantothenate effective in rheumatoid arthritis. Has been used to decrease allergic skin reactions in children and to overcome excess mucous secretion in respiratory allergies in adults.

---

**papaya,** also known as pawpaw. Rich source of carotene at 500µg per 100g in the canned fruit; no detectable vitamin E. B vitamins present are (in mg per 100g): thiamine 0.02; riboflavin 0.02; nicotinic acid 0.2; pantothenic acid 0.2. Vitamin C content of 15mg per 100g.

---

**para-aminobenzoic acid,** member of the vitamin B complex but not a true vitamin for man. Known also as PABA, vitamin Bx, bacterial vitamin H, anti-gray-hair factor. Growth factor for bacteria that is blocked by sulphonamide drugs, first reported by D. D. Woods at Oxford in 1942. PABA is present as part of the structure of folic acid but no evidence that humans can make folic acid from it. Likely that intestinal bacteria can, but body unable to utilize the folic acid produced.

*Richest food sources* are: liver, eggs, molasses, brewer's yeast, wheat germ. Few figures are available but baker's yeast contains 6mg per kg; brewer's yeast up to 100mg per kg.

*Stability* in food processing unknown.

*Functions in man* not known. *Deficiency in man* gives no specific symptoms.

*Functions in animals* in synthesis of body protein and in red blood cell production, possibly after conversion to folic acid. Helps utilization of pantothenic acid. May act as skin cancer preventative. *Deficiency in animals* causes anemia, premature graying of hair.

*Recommended dietary intakes* not set by any authority. *Supplementation* restricted to maximum potency of 30mg per unit dose in the UK.

*Toxicity* is low but high intakes can cause nausea, vomiting, itch, skin rash and liver damage. *Contra-indicated* when on sulphonamide treatment.

*Therapy* with oral PABA in vitiligo. As lotion or cream is effective as sunscreen agent to prevent sunburn. May also prevent skin cancer. Has been used in digestive disorders, nervousness, depression.

---

**para-amino salicylic acid,** anti-tuberculosis drug. Impairs absorption of vitamins A, D, E and K and of $B_{12}$.

---

**paralytic ileus,** *see* surgery.

---

**paresthesia,** tingling or pricking feeling or sometimes numbness in the skin. Symptom of multiple sclerosis, nerve disease, blood-vessel disease. Relieved by pyridoxine (50mg daily).

---

**Parkinson's disease,** a chronic disease of the central nervous system characterized by slowness and poorness of purposeful movement, rigid muscles and tremor. Also known as Parkinsonism, shaking palsy.

Drug *levodopa,* used to bring symptomatic relief, is neutralized by pyridoxine; therefore supplements of vitamin should *not* be taken while on drug. Side-effects of levodopa may be lessened by taking vitamin C (500 to 1000mg daily).

---

**parsley,** in raw state, rich source of carotene, providing average 7.0mg per 100g. Vitamin E content is 1.8mg per 100g. B vitamins present are (in mg per 100g): thiamine 0.15; riboflavin 0.30; nicotinic acid 1.8; pyridoxine 0.20; pantothenic acid 0.30. Contains no folic acid and only 0.4µg per 100g biotin. Excellent source of vitamin C at average 150mg per 100g.

---

**parsnips,** losses of all water-soluble vitamins present on boiling. Traces only of carotene with concentration of vitamin E 1.0mg per 100g. Levels of B vitamins are (in mg per 100g), raw figures first: thiamine 0.10, 0.07; riboflavin 0.08, 0.06; nicotinic acid 1.3, 0.9; pyridoxine 0.10, 0.06; pantothenic acid 0.50, 0.35. Folic acid level reduces from 67 to 30μg per 100g on boiling; traces only of biotin present. Vitamin C content drops from 15 to 10mg per 100g on boiling.

---

**passion fruit,** good source of vitamin C with some B vitamins present in raw, edible portion. Carotene content is 10μg per 100g; vitamin E has not been detected. B vitamins present are (in mg per 100g): thiamine, traces only; riboflavin 0.10; nicotinic acid 1.9. Good source of vitamin C at 20mg per 100g.

---

**Pauling, Linus,** American scientist, twice winner of Nobel Prize, who coined the phrase "orthomolecular psychiatry" in "the treatment of mental disease by the provision of the optimum molecular environment of the mind, especially the optimum concentrations of substances usually present in the human body." Introduced concept of high-potency vitamin C to prevent and treat respiratory infections. Founded Institute of Orthomolecular Medicine, Menlo Park, Stanford, California, USA.

---

**peaches,** in the raw state are a rich source of carotene with useful levels of B vitamins and vitamin C. Canned peaches show lower concentrations of all vitamins compared with the fresh type. Carotene contents of fresh, edible portion and canned variety respectively (in μg per 100g) are 500 and 250; vitamin E has not been detected. B vitamins present are (in mg per 100g) for raw, edible portion and canned variety respectively: thiamine 0.02, 0.01; riboflavin 0.05, 0.02; nicotinic acid 1.0, 0.6; pyridoxine 0.02, 0.02; pantothenic acid 0.15, 0.05. Similar folic acid levels at 3μg per 100g; similar biotin levels at 0.2μg per 100g. Vitamin C reduced from 8mg per 100g in raw, edible portion to 4mg per 100g in canned variety. *See also* dried peaches.

---

**peanut butter,** supplies good quantities of vitamin E and the B vitamins. Vitamin E content is 7.6mg per 100g. B vitamins present are (in mg per 100g): thiamine 0.17; riboflavin 0.10; nicotinic acid 19.9; pyridoxine 0.50;

pantothenic acid 2.1. Folic acid level is 53μg per 100g. Traces only of vitamin C. Similar vitamin contents in both smooth and crunchy peanut butter.

---

**peanuts,** kernels supply good quantities of vitamin E and B vitamins. Some B vitamins reduced when peanuts are roasted and salted. Vitamin E contents of fresh kernels and those that have been roasted and salted are identical at 16.9mg per 100g. B vitamins present (in mg per 100g), for fresh kernels and those that have been roasted and salted respectively, are: thiamine 0.90, 0.23; riboflavin 0.10, 0.10; nicotinic acid 21.3, 21.3; pyridoxine 0.50, 0.40; pantothenic acid 2.7, 2.1. Folic acid level in fresh kernels is 110μg per 100g, but is not detectable in the roasted and salted variety. Traces only of vitamin C in fresh and roasted peanuts.

---

**pears,** edible portion of eating variety has poor content of all vitamins either in raw state or as canned variety. Loss of B vitamins and vitamin C during canning. Carotene content is 10μg per 100g; traces only of vitamin E in both eating and canned pears. B vitamins present are (in mg per 100g), for eating and canned pears respectively: thiamine 0.03, 0.01; riboflavin 0.03, 0.01; nicotinic acid 0.3, 0.2; pyridoxine 0.02, 0.01; pantothenic acid 0.07, 0.02. Folic acid content is 11μg per 100g for fresh, edible portion of fruit and 5μg per 100g for canned fruit. Biotin is 1μg per 100g and a trace respectively. Vitamin C is reduced from 3mg to 1mg per 100g when fruit is canned.

*Cooking* variety have similar concentrations of vitamins to eating pears with only slight losses on stewing, with and without sugar. Carotene levels for raw, cooking pears, stewed without sugar and stewed with sugar respectively, are (in μg per 100g) 10, 9 and 8. Traces only of vitamin E. B vitamins present are (in mg per 100g), for raw, cooking pears, stewed without sugar and stewed with sugar respectively: thiamine 0.03, 0.03, 0.02; riboflavin 0.03, 0.03, 0.02; nicotinic acid 0.2, 0.2, 0.2; pyridoxine 0.02, 0.02, 0.02; pantothenic acid 0.07, 0.05, 0.05. Folic acid levels are respectively 11, 5 and 5μg per 100g; biotin levels are stable at 0.1μg per 100g respectively for the three states of cooking pears.

---

**peas,** when boiled, fresh peas lose substantial quantities of B vitamins and vitamin C. Fat-soluble vitamins are unaffected. Concentrations of carotene and vitamin E (in mg per 100g) in both raw and boiled fresh peas are 0.3 and 0.9mg respectively. Levels of B vitamins (in mg per 100g) are, for raw and boiled peas respectively: thiamine 0.32, 0.25; riboflavin 0.15, 0.11; nicotinic acid 3.4, 2.3; pyridoxine 0.16, 0.10; pantothenic acid 0.75, 0.32. Folic acid levels are not known, but those of biotin are 0.5 and 0.4µg per 100g for raw and boiled peas. Vitamin C level is reduced from 25 to 15mg per 100g on boiling fresh peas. *See also* canned peas, dried peas and frozen peas.

**pecan nuts,**　good source of carotene at 80µg per 100g. Vitamin E level is 1.5mg per 100g. B vitamins present are (in mg per 100g): thiamine 0.86; riboflavin 0.13; nicotinic acid 0.9; pyridoxine 0.19. Vitamin C content is 2mg per 100g.

**pellagra,**　specific disease associated with deficiency of nicotinic acid and characterized by skin, mucous membrane, central nervous system and gastro-intestinal symptoms. Symptoms may appear alone or in combination. Treatment is 300 to 1000mg nicotinamide daily in divided doses.

Similar disease in dogs known as canine black tongue.

**penicillamine,**　anti-arthritic drug. Enhances excretion of pyridoxine.

**pentamidine isethionate,**　anti-protozoal drug. Impairs folic acid utilization.

**peppers,**　good source of carotene that is stable to boiling. Excellent source of vitamin C but poor source of B vitamins. Average carotene content in both raw and boiled green peppers is 200µg (range 60-1000) per 100g. Contribute 0.8mg vitamin E per 100g either cooked or raw. B vitamins are reduced on boiling green peppers, with concentrations (in mg per 100g) of, raw figures first: thiamine 0.01, trace; riboflavin 0.03, 0.02; nicotinic acid 0.9, 0.8; pyridoxine 0.17, 0.14; pantothenic acid 0.23, 0.16. Folic acid levels are stable at 11µg per 100g. Vitamin C content reduced from 100 to 60mg per 100g on boiling.

**pernicious anemia,**　particular type of anemia, also known as

Addisonian anemia, characterized by non-specific symptoms, loss of appetite, constipation alternating with diarrhea, and vague abdominal pains. More specific is "burning of the tongue" or glossitis. Considerable weight loss. Later there is nervous involvement with tingling in the extremities, irritability, depression, delirium, and paranoia. Loss of sensation in lower extremities.

Only treatment is vitamin $B_{12}$ by injection, which continues throughout life.

---

**Pfieffer, Carl, C.,** American doctor who as Director of the Brain Bio Center, Princeton, New Jersey, USA, has utilized vitamin therapy in treating many diseases including those associated with mental disturbances.

---

**PGA,** *see* folic acid.

---

**phagocytes,** white blood cells that engulf and destroy invading microorganisms. *See* leucocytes.

---

**pheneturide,** anti-convulsant drug. Reduces conversion of vitamin D to 25-hydroxy vitamin D.

---

**phenformin,** anti-diabetic drug. Prevents absorption of vitamin $B_{12}$.

---

**phenylbutazone,** anti-arthritic drug. Impairs folic acid utilization.

---

**phenytoin,** anti-convulsant drug. Reduces body levels of folic acid and 25-hydroxy vitamin D.

---

**phlebitis,** presence of a thrombosis in a vein that causes painful, tender and swollen lump, usually in the leg. Daily intake of 200IU vitamin E believed to prevent condition. Treatment needs daily intake of at least 600IU vitamin E.

---

**phosphorus,** essential mineral that, in the form of phosphate, is needed to activate most of the B vitamins. As adenosine triphosphate (ATP) is the hub of energy production in the body.

---

**phylloquinone,** *see* K vitamin.

---

**phytomenadione,** *see* K vitamin.

---

**phytonadione,** *see* K vitamin.

---

**piccalilli,** vegetable relish. Provides only thiamine, riboflavin and nicotinic acid at levels of 0.16, 0.01 and 0.4mg per 100g respectively. Traces of vitamin C present.

---

**pine nuts,** carotene content is 18μg per 100g. B vitamins present are (in mg per 100g): thiamine 1.28; riboflavin 0.23; nicotinic acid 4.5. Other vitamins have not been measured.

---

**pineapple,** some losses in all vitamins present when raw, edible portion of fruit is canned. Fresh pineapple is good source of vitamin C. Carotene content is 60 and 40μg per 100g for fresh and canned varieties respectively. B vitamins present are (in mg per 100g), for fresh, edible portion and canned pineapple respectively: thiamine 0.08, 0.05; riboflavin 0.02, 0.02; nicotinic acid 0.3, 0.2; pyridoxine 0.09, 0.07; pantothenic acid 0.16, 0.10. Folic acid levels are 11 and 2μg per 100g for fresh, edible portion and canned pineapple respectively; traces only of biotin. Vitamin C content is 25mg (range 20-40mg) per 100g for fresh pineapple and 12mg per 100g for the canned fruit.

---

**pineapple juice,** when canned, provides some vitamin C and B vitamins with carotene but no detectable vitamin E. Carotene content is 40μg per 100g. B vitamins present are (in mg per 100g): thiamine 0.05; riboflavin 0.02; nicotinic acid 0.3; pyridoxine 0.10; pantothenic acid 0.10. Folic acid level is 2µg per 100g; biotin was not detected. Vitamin C content is 8mg per 100g.

**pistachio nuts,**   very good source of carotene at 138µg per 100g. B vitamins present are thiamine (0.67mg per 100g) and nicotinic acid (1.4mg per 100g). Other vitamins have not been measured.

**plantain,**   carotene present is stable to boiling and frying and contributes 60µg per 100g. Vitamin E is absent. Low levels of B vitamins that are less affected by frying than boiling. Figures (in mg per 100g) for raw, boiled and fried respectively, are: thiamine 0.05, trace, 0.11; riboflavin 0.05, 0.01, 0.02; nicotinic acid 0.9, 0.5, 0.8; pyridoxine 0.50, 0.30, 1.0; pantothenic acid 0.37, 0.26, 0.73. Folic acid levels are respectively 16, 18, 37µg per 100g. The higher levels in the fried plant are because the plantain is fried only when ripe. Vitamin C contents are 20, 3 and 12mg per 100g respectively.

**plums,**   Victoria dessert, edible portion only supply good quantities of carotene with low levels of other vitamins. Carotene content is 220µg per 100g; plus 0.7mg vitamin E per 100g. B vitamins present are (in mg per 100g): thiamine 0.05; riboflavin 0.03; nicotinic acid 0.6; pyridoxine 0.05; pantothenic acid 0.15. Folic acid level only 3µg per 100g with traces only of biotin. Vitamin C content only 3mg per 100g edible portion.

  *Cooking* variety provide good quantities of carotene with levels of B vitamins and vitamin C comparable to eating plums. Slight losses only on stewing, without and with sugar. Carotene contents are (in µg per 100g) for raw cooking plums stewed without sugar and stewed with sugar respectively, 220, 180 and 170. B vitamins present are (in mg per 100g), for raw, edible plums, stewed without sugar and stewed with sugar respectively: thiamine 0.05, 0.04, 0.04; riboflavin 0.03, 0.03, 0.02; nicotinic acid 0.6, 0.6, 0.5; pyridoxine 0.05, 0.03, 0.03; pantothenic acid 0.15, 0.12, 0.11. Folic acid levels are (in µg per 100g) respectively 3, 1, 1; traces only of biotin. Vitamin C contents are respectively 3, 3 and 2mg per 100g.

**pollution,**   atmospheric produced by carbon monoxide and lead from exhaust fumes, ozone, nitrogen dioxide, sulphur dioxide and dust.

  Vitamin C protects against carbon monoxide and lead. Vitamin E protects against ozone and other oxidizers. Also protects vitamin A against destruction by ozone and nitrogen dioxide. Polluted atmosphere prevents ultra-violet light reaching skin so vitamin D is not synthesized and dietary intake must be increased.

**polymixin,** antibiotic. Prevents formation of vitamin K by intestinal bacteria.

**polyunsaturated fatty acids,** originally called vitamin F applied to linoleic, linolenic and arachidonic acids. Now unofficially applied to linoleic acid alone since this is the precursor of the other two in the body. Known also as PUFA, essential fatty acids, EFA. Essentially first demonstrated by G. O. Burr and M. M. Burr in 1929 who found those acids needed by rats for health and survival. Main sources of linoleic acid are vegetable and seed oils. Recently PUFA from fish body oils called EPA (eicosapentaenoic acid) and DHA (docosahexaenoic acid) found to be essential.

*Richest food sources of linoleic acid* (in grams per 100g) are: oil of evening primrose (72.70); safflower oil (71.63); soybean oil (49.66); corn oil (47.75); wheat germ oil (41.54); peanut oil (27.70); olive oil (10.51). Oil of evening primrose contains in addition to linoleic acid, gammalinolenic acid (average 8 per cent).

*Functions* are constituents of cell membranes and myelin sheath of nerves; precursors of hormones called prostaglandins; constituents of cholesteryl esters; constituents of triglycerides (body fats).

*Deficiency* in animals and man causes mild skin complaints including scaly dermatitis. May cause infantile eczema.

*Recommended dietary intake* — none laid down by any authority but many recommended that most of fat intakes (25-35 per cent of calories) should be as PUFA oils.

*Therapy* has proved beneficial in: mild skin complaints; in atopic eczema; in infantile eczema; in premenstrual tension; in multiple sclerosis; in thrombosis prevention; in reducing high blood cholesterol levels. EPA and DHA appear beneficial in: increasing blood clotting time (i.e., thinning the blood); in angina pectoris; in reducing high blood fat concentrations; in preventing thrombosis formation.

**PP factor,** *see* nicotinic acid.

**pomegranate,**   both raw, edible portion of fruit and the juice contain only small quantities of the B vitamins plus vitamin C. Those present are (in mg per 100g): thiamine 0.02; riboflavin 0.03; nicotinic acid 0.2; vitamin C 8. Figures apply only to fruit and to juice.

---

**pork,**   all cuts when cooked supply only traces of vitamin A, D and carotene. Vitamin E ranges from 0.01 to 0.12mg per 100g. Poor source of folic acid and biotin. Other B vitamins (in mg per 100g) are in the range: thiamine 0.45-0.88; riboflavin 0.11-0.35; nicotinic acid 6.2-13.6; pyridoxine 0.23-0.41; pantothenic acid 0.5-1.3; (in $\mu$g per 100g) vitamin $B_{12}$ 1-2; folic acid 3-7.

Higher potencies associated with leaner cuts. Completely devoid of vitamin C. *See also* Meats: Cooking losses.

---

**port,**   a fortified wine providing very little quantities of vitamins. Trace only of carotene. B vitamins present are (in mg per 100ml): thiamine, trace; riboflavin 0.01; nicotinic acid 0.06; pyridoxine 0.01; vitamin $B_{12}$, trace. Trace only of folic acid. Completely devoid of vitamin C.

---

**potatoes,**   all potatoes, old and new, cooked in every way, contain only traces of carotene and 0.1mg vitamin E per 100g. Poor source of B vitamins but usually regarded as an important source of vitamin C in the Western diet.

*Raw* potatoes when old contain the following B vitamins (in mg per 100g): thiamine 0.11; riboflavin 0.04; nicotinic acid 1.7; pyridoxine 0.25; pantothenic acid 0.30. Folic acid content is 14$\mu$g per 100g; biotin present only in traces. Vitamin C levels vary from 8 to 20mg per 100g depending on age of potato.

*Boiled old* potatoes when eaten plain or mashed lose some of their B vitamins which can be recovered by utilizing water in which they were boiled. Concentrations in boiled and mashed are identical and are (in mg per 100g): thiamine 0.08; riboflavin 0.03; nicotinic acid 1.1; pyridoxine 0.18; pantothenic acid 0.20. Contribute 10$\mu$g per 100g of folic acid but only traces of biotin. Level of vitamin C in range 4 to 14mg per 100g.

*Baked* potatoes contain the following B vitamins, with and without skins respectively (in mg per 100g): thiamine 0.08, 0.10; riboflavin 0.03, 0.04; nicotinic acid 1.5, 1.8; pyridoxine 0.14, 0.18; pantothenic acid 0.16, 0.20. Folic acid concentrations are 8 and 10$\mu$g per 100g with and without skins respectively. Levels of vitamin C in ranges 5-16 and 4-13mg per 100g for baked potatoes without and with skins respectively.

*Roasted* potatoes lose less B vitamins than the boiled variety. Final concentrations (in mg per 100g) are: thiamine 0.10; riboflavin 0.04; nicotinic acid 1.9; pyridoxine 0.18; pantothenic acid 0.20. Folic acid concentration is 7µg per 100g. Levels of vitamin C in range 5-16mg per 100g.

*Fries* have similar concentrations of B vitamins to roasted potatoes with the following differences: nicotinic acid 2.1mg per 100g; folic acid 10µg per 100g. Levels of vitamin C in range 5-16mg per 100g.

*Chips* are better sources of B vitamins and particularly vitamin E. The latter is due to the vitamin contributed by the cooking oil. Vitamin E content is 6.1mg per 100g. Levels of B vitamins are (in mg per 100g): thiamine 0.19; riboflavin 0.07; nicotinic acid 6.1; pyridoxine 0.89; pantothenic acid 0.20. Folic acid content is 20µg per 100g. Good source of vitamin C at 17mg per 100g.

*See also* dried potatoes, frozen fries and new potatoes.

**precursors,** substances that occur in food that are not vitamins in their own right but can give rise to vitamins in the body or during cooking processes.

Examples are: *carotenes,* some of which are converted to vitamin A in the intestine and liver; *L-tryptophane,* an essential amino acid of food proteins, converted to nicotinic acid in the liver under the influence of thiamine, riboflavin, pyridoxine and biotin; *niacytin,* a bound form of nicotinic acid that occurs in corn and other cereals, unavailable to the body unless cooked under alkaline conditions which liberates nicotinic acid; *7-dehydrocholesterol* in the skin, converted to vitamin D by the action of sunlight or particular wavelengths of ultra-violet light. *Vitamin D* itself is inactive but is a precursor of 25-hydroxy D and 1,25-dihydroxy D which are its active forms in the body.

**pregnancy,** all authorities recognize that all vitamins and some minerals must be increased in dietary intake but no agreement on extent of increase. Blood levels of vitamin A, nicotinamide, pyridoxine, vitamin $B_{12}$ and ascorbic acid markedly decreased in pregnant women suggesting all should be supplemented. Some evidence that low vitamin levels may lead to some birth defects in offspring. Daily supplementation with good all-round multivitamin preparation recommended throughout pregnancy since availability from diet highly unlikely. Folic acid is a special case. Amounts required are above level allowed to be sold to public so must be obtained from practitioner.

---

**prickly heat,** known also as milaria, characterized by small pimples on skin surface that irritate, causes scratching and eventual bleeding of the affected area. Induced by retained sweat. Treated and prevented by daily dose of 1000mg vitamin C for adult weighing 150lbs, proportionally less for children depending on weight.

---

**primidone,** anti-convulsant drug. Reduces conversion of vitamin D to 25-hydroxy vitamin D.

---

**processed meats,** such as canned meat, pastes, sausages, beefburgers and pies all supply significantly less vitamins than the meat from which they were made. Reduced levels are due to processing losses and dilution of the meat with fat and flour.

---

**prostaglandins,** hormones produced within the body that control many metabolic processes. All prostaglandins are made from polyunsaturated fatty acids, linoleic acid and alpha linolenic acid, each acid producing a separate series of prostaglandins.

Prostaglandins can make blood thick, so increasing chances of thrombosis, or thin, preventing thrombosis. Production of "thinning" prostaglandins are stimulated by vitamin E. PUFA from fish body oils, called EPA and DHA, also thin the blood, reducing its ability to form thrombosis because they are precursors of "thinning" prostaglandins.

---

**prostate problems,** usually due to inflammation or enlargement. Supplemented needs include PUFA (safflower oil, oil of evening primrose), 3g daily, plus mineral zinc, 20mg daily.

---

**protein,** nutrient that is supplied in the diet, digested to amino acids and absorbed in the gastro-intestinal tract then rebuilt by the body into its own proteins required for growth and repairing of body cells, tissues, muscles and organs.

*Synthesis* of body proteins requires vitamin A: high protein intakes require concomitant vitamin A intake. Also pyridoxine. *Blood clotting proteins* require vitamin K for synthesis. *Nucleoproteins* are complexes of protein and nucleic acids and need vitamin $B_{12}$ for synthesis. *See* nucleic acids.

**prunes,** these are dried plums so most vitamins are present in higher concentration than in fresh fruit. Vitamin C virtually disappears during drying process. Some losses during stewing process both without and with sugar. Carotene content, for raw, edible portion, stewed without sugar and stewed with sugar, respectively, is 1000, 510 and 470μg per 100g; vitamin E is negligible. B vitamins present (in mg per 100g) for raw, edible portion, stewed without sugar and stewed with sugar, respectively, are: thiamine 0.10, 0.04, 0.04; riboflavin 0.20, 0.09, 0.09; nicotinic acid 1.9, 1.0, 0.9; pyridoxine 0.24, 0.10, 0.10; pantothenic acid 0.46, 0.21, 0.20. Folic acid levels are (in μg per 100g) 4, trace, trace, respectively; traces only of biotin. Traces only of vitamin C present.

**psoriasis,** common chronic and recurrent skin disease characterized by dry, silvery, scaling eruptions and plaques of various sizes due to overproduction of epithelial cells. Has been treated with oral and topical (applied to skin) vitamin A, retinoic acid and synthetic vitamin A derivatives.

**pteroyglutamic acid,** *see* folic acid.

**pteroyl monoglutamic acid,** *see* folic acid.

**pudding,** *milk,* supplies all vitamins (in mg per 100g): vitamin A 0.3; carotene 0.02; thiamine 0.04; riboflavin 0.14; nicotinic acid 1.1; pyridoxine 0.05; folic acid 0.004; pantothenic acid 0.3; biotin 0.002; vitamin $B_{12}$ trace; vitamin C trace; vitamin E 0.1; vitamin D 0.02μg.

*Yorkshire,* supplies all vitamins (in mg per 100g): vitamin A 0.04; carotene 0.06; thiamine 0.17; riboflavin 0.05; nicotinic acid 2.2; pyridoxine 0.07; pantothenic acid 0.4; biotin 0.005; vitamin $B_{12}$ trace; vitamin C trace;

vitamin E 0.3; vitamin D 0.26µg.

---

**PUFA,** *see* polyunsaturated fatty acids.

---

**pumpkin,** good source of carotene but little in the way of B vitamins. Vitamin E is virtually absent. Supplies 1.5mg carotene per 100g (range 0.7-2.0). B vitamins present are (in mg per 100g): thiamine 0.04; riboflavin 0.04; nicotinic acid 0.5; pyridoxine 0.06; pantothenic acid 0.40. Quantity of folic acid (in µg per 100g) present is 13 and that of biotin is 0.4. Vitamin C content is 5mg per 100g.

---

**purpura,** hemorrhages under the skin that occur without definite cause or due to slight injury. Has been treated with oral vitamin E, 400-600IU daily, until purpura disappears. *See also* bruises.

---

**pyridoxal,** *see* $B_6$ vitamin.

---

**pyridoxamine,** *see* $B_6$ vitamin.

---

**pyridoxine,** *see* $B_6$ vitamin.

---

**pyrimethamine,** antimalarial drug. Impairs folic acid utilization.

# Q

---

**quinces,** the raw variety provide good quantities of vitamin C with small amounts of some B vitamins. Traces only of carotene with no detectable vitamin E. B vitamins present (in mg per 100g) are: thiamine 0.02; riboflavin

0.02; nicotinic acid 0.2. Vitamin C content is 15mg per 100g edible portion.

# R

**radishes,**   virtually devoid of carotene and vitamin E. Poor source of B vitamins but supplies useful quantities of vitamin C. B vitamins present are (in mg per 100g): thiamine 0.04; riboflavin 0.02; nicotinic acid 0.4; pyridoxine 0.10; pantothenic acid 0.18. Contribute 24μg folic acid per 100g but no biotin. Vitamin C content is 25mg per 100g (range 10-35).

**raisins,**   these are dried grapes that are more concentrated in vitamins than the raw, fresh fruit, apart from vitamin C. Carotene content is 30μg per 100g; vitamin E has not been detected. B vitamins present are (in mg per 100g): thiamine 0.10; riboflavin 0.08; nicotinic acid 0.6; pyridoxine 0.30; pantothenic acid 0.10. Folic acid level is 4μg per 100g; biotin is absent. Completely devoid of vitamin C.

**raspberries,**   good source of vitamin C with some carotene and B vitamins and useful quantities of vitamin E. Most of the vitamins are retained when the fruit is stewed but some losses occur when it is canned. Carotene contents are for the raw fruit, stewed without sugar, stewed with sugar and canned: 80, 85, 75μg per 100g respectively. Vitamin E is stable at 4.5mg per 100g in all four forms. B vitamins present are (in mg per 100g), for the raw fruit, stewed without sugar, stewed with sugar and canned, respectively: thiamine 0.02, 0.02, 0.02, 0.01; riboflavin 0.03 for all four forms; nicotinic acid 0.5, 0.5, 0.5, 0.4; pyridoxine 0.06, 0.05, 0.05, 0.04; pantothenic acid 0.24, 0.23, 0.21, 0.17. Folic acid appears to be absent but biotin levels are respectively 1.9, 2.0, 1.8 and 1.6μg per 100g. Vitamin C contents are (in mg per 100g), for the four forms of raspberries: 25 (range 14-35), 23, 22 and 7 respectively.

*Frozen* raspberries have similar contents of carotene and all vitamins to the fresh fruit, but the vitamin C level is reduced to 20mg per 100g.

# Table 18: Recommended dietary intakes for adults

| | | Ca | Cz | Dn | FDR | Fl | GDR | H | I | Ne | No | Po | Ro | Sp | Sw | UK | USA | USSR | WHO/FAO |
|---|---|---|---|---|---|---|---|---|---|---|---|---|---|---|---|---|---|---|---|
| VITAMIN A | Female | 800 | 1000 | 800 | 900 | 750 | 900 | 750 | 750 | 450 | 750 | 1500 | 1500 | 750 | 900 | 750 | 800 | 1500 | 750 |
| µg | Male | 1000 | | | 1000 | | | | | | | | | | | | 1000 | | |
| THIAMINE | Female | 1.4 | 0.9 | 1.0 | 1.4 | 0.8 | 1.5 | 1.1 | 0.9 | 0.8 | 1.0 | 1.4 | 1.8 | 0.9 | 1.0 | 0.9 | 1.0 | 1.5 | 0.9 |
| mg | Male | 1.0 | 1.1 | 1.4 | 1.6 | 0.9 | 1.6 | | 1.2 | 1.0 | 1.4 | 1.7 | 2.1 | 1.2 | 1.4 | 1.1 | 1.4 | 1.8 | 1.2 |
| RIBOFLAVIN | Female | 1.7 | 1.4 | 1.2 | 1.6 | 1.3 | 1.5 | 1.5 | 1.2 | 1.2 | 1.5 | 1.4 | 2.0 | 1.3 | 1.5 | 1.3 | 1.2 | 2.0 | 1.3 |
| mg | Male | 1.2 | 1.6 | 1.6 | 2.0 | 1.4 | 1.6 | | 1.6 | 1.4 | 1.7 | 1.7 | 2.4 | 1.8 | 1.7 | 1.7 | 1.6 | 2.4 | 1.8 |
| PYRIDOXINE | Female | 2.0 | 1.8 | 2.0 | 1.6 | – | – | – | – | – | – | 2.0 | 1.7 | – | – | – | 2.0 | 1.8 | – |
| mg | Male | 1.5 | 1.9 | | 1.8 | | | | | | | | | | | | | 2.1 | |
| PANTOTHENIC ACID mg | | – | – | – | 8.0 | – | – | – | – | – | – | – | – | – | – | – | – | – | – |
| VITAMIN B₁₂ µg | | 3.0 | – | 3.0 | 5.0 | – | – | – | 2.0 | – | – | 5.0 | – | 2.0 | – | – | 3.0 | – | 2.0 |
| VITAMIN C | Female | 30 | 50 | 45 | 75 | 30 | 70 | 30 | 45 | 50 | 30 | 70 | 75 | 30 | 55 | 30 | 45 | 64 | 30 |
| mg | Male | | | | | | | | | | | 75 | 85 | | 60 | | | 75 | |
| BIOFLAVONOIDS | Female | – | – | – | – | – | – | – | – | – | – | 14 | 16 | – | – | – | | 17 | – |
| mg | Male | | | | | | | | | | | 17 | 18 | | | | | 20 | |
| VITAMIN E | Female | 8 | 10 | 12 | 12 | – | – | – | – | – | – | 25 | 10 | – | – | – | 12 | – | – |
| mg | Male | 6 | 12 | 15 | | | | | | | | 30 | | | | | 15 | | |
| VITAMIN D µg | | 2.5 | 2.5 | 2.5 | 2.5 | 2.5 | 2.5 | 2.5 | 2.5 | 2.5 | 2.5 | 2.5 | 2.5 | 2.5 | 2.5 | 2.5 | 5.0 / 7.0 | – | 2.5 |

Key:
Ca: Canada
Cz: Czechoslovakia
Dn: Denmark
FDR: West Germany
Fl: Finland
GDR: East Germany
H: Hungary
I: Italy
Ne: Netherlands
No: Norway
Po: Poland
Ro: Romania
Sp: Spain
Sw: Sweden
UK: United Kingdom
USA: United States of America
USSR: Russia
FAO/ Food and Agricultural Organization
WHO: World Health Organization

154

**RDA,**   recommended daily allowance. *See* recommended dietary intakes.

---

**recommended dietary intakes,**   known in USA as recommended daily allowances (RDA). Daily minimum requirements of vitamins needed to prevent symptoms of deficiency disease but not necessarily sufficient to maintain optimum health. Safety factors added to average minimum requirements to deal with three variables:

1.   to take account of individual variations in requirements — safety factor covers 95 per cent of population.
2.   to take account of possible increases caused by minor stresses of life but extra needs during infections, injuries and other illnesses are ignored.
3.   to take account of different availability of vitamins in various foods.

Figures vary among countries reflecting variation in how they are arrived at. Also number of vitamins with recommended intakes differ amongst several authorities. For figures *see* Table 18.

---

**regional enteritis,**   *see* Crohn's disease.

---

**red cabbage,**   *in raw state* is poor source of carotene at only 20μg per 100g and of vitamin E at 0.2mg per 100g. B vitamins present are (in mg per 100g): thiamine 0.06; riboflavin 0.05; nicotinic acid 0.6; pyridoxine 0.21; pantothenic acid 0.32. Folic acid is present in reasonable amounts (90μg per 100g) but trace only of biotin. Good source of vitamin C at 55mg per 100g.

---

**red kidney beans,**   when raw are virtually devoid of fat-soluble vitamins. B vitamins present in good quantities are (in mg per 100g): thiamine 0.54; riboflavin 0.18; nicotinic acid 5.5; pyridoxine 0.44; pantothenic acid 0.50. Good source of folic acid at 130μg per 100g. Negligible vitamin C content.

---

**red currants,**   less rich in vitamin C than black variety but B vitamin levels are similar. Lower concentrations also of carotene and vitamin E. Supply 70μg per 100g of carotene in raw state, reduced to 55μg when stewed. Vitamin E levels stable at 0.1mg per 100g. B vitamins present are (in mg per 100g), for raw and stewed fruit respectively: thiamine 0.04, 0.03;

riboflavin 0.06, 0.05; nicotinic acid 0.3, 0.2; pyridoxine 0.05, 0.03; pantothenic acid 0.06, 0.05. Biotin levels are 2.6 and 2.0µg per 100g respectively for raw and stewed fruit. Folic acid is absent. Good source of vitamin C at levels of 40mg per 100g for raw fruit, reduced to 30mg on stewing.

**retinal,**   vitamin A aldehyde, retinaldehyde, active form of vitamin A in sight process.

**retinene,**   old name for retinal.

**retinoic acid,**   vitamin A acid, active form of vitamin A in growth. Used on skin in treating skin complaints including skin cancer.

**retinoid,**   term to describe vitamin A and its derivatives both natural and synthetic.

**retinol,**   *see* vitamin A.

**retrolental fibroplasia,**   eye problem in premature babies. *See* oxygen and vitamin E.

**rheumatism,**   general term indicating diseases of muscle, tendon, joint, bone or nerve resulting in discomfort and disability. Often used to include rheumatoid arthritis, osteoarthritis, spondylitis, bursitis, fibrositis, myositis, lumbago, sciatica and gout. Vitamin therapy as for rheumatoid arthritis. *See* gout.

**rheumatoid arthritis,**   *see* arthritis.

**rhubarb,**   supplies some carotene, vitamin E and vitamin C with small amounts of B vitamins. Carotene contents of raw rhubarb, that stewed without sugar and that stewed with sugar, respectively are 60, 55 and 50µg per 100g. Vitamin E is stable at 0.2mg per 100g for all three forms. B vitamins present are (in mg per 100g), for raw, stewed without sugar and stewed with sugar respectively: thiamine 0.10, trace, trace; riboflavin 0.03, 0.03, 0.03; nicotinic acid 0.4, 0.4, 0.4; pyridoxine 0.03, 0.02, 0.02; pantothenic acid 0.08, 0.06, 0.05. Folic acid levels are 8, 4 and 4µg per 100g respectively for the three forms of fruit. Biotin has not been detected. Vitamin C contents are 10, 8 and 7mg per 100g respectively.

*Canned* rhubarb has similar levels of vitamins to those of the stewed fruit with the exception of vitamin C which is only 1mg per 100g.

---

**riboflavin(e),**   *see* B$_2$ vitamin.

---

**ribonucleic acid (RNA),**   *see* nucleic acids.

---

**rice,**   *polished, raw* rice is useful source of B vitamins, providing (in mg per 100g): thiamine 0.08; riboflavin 0.03; nicotinic acid 3.0; pyridoxine 0.30; folic acid 0.029; pantothenic acid 0.6; biotin 0.003; vitamin E 0.6. Main source of B vitamins when rice is part of staple diet.

*Boiled,* is much reduced in B vitamins but losses leached into water can be recovered and used. Provides (in mg per 100g): thiamine 0.01; riboflavin 0.01; nicotinic acid 0.8; pyridoxine 0.05; folic acid 0.006; pantothenic acid 0.2; biotin 0.001; vitamin E 0.1.

---

**rickets,**   disease in children characterized by lack of mineralization of bones and due to deficiency of vitamin D.

*Symptoms* are restlessness, poor ability to sleep and constant head movement. Infants do not sit, crawl or walk early and closing of the soft joints in head bones is delayed. Weight-bearing eventually bends the bones causing bow legs, knock-knees in the legs and pigeon breast.

*Therapy* is doses up to 20 000IU daily with calcium and phosphorus.

---

**Robbins, R. C.,**   American scientist at the University of Florida who has carried out comprehensive studies on the bioflavonoids and their relationship to treatment of disease.

---

**roe,** *hard variety* is useful source of vitamins. Concentrations of vitamins A and D are 140μg and 2.0μg per 100g respectively. Good source of vitamin E at 6.9mg per 100g. B vitamins present (in mg per 100g) are: thiamine 1.5; riboflavin 1.0; nicotinic acid 6.0; pyridoxine 0.32; pantothenic acid 3.0. Excellent source of vitamin $B_{12}$ at 10μg per 100g; and biotin at 15μg per 100g. One of the best seafood sources of vitamin C at 30mg per 100g.

*Soft variety* is less rich in vitamins. Fat soluble not detected. B vitamins (in mg per 100g) present are: thiamine 0.20; riboflavin 0.50; nicotinic acid 4.5; pantothenic acid 0.49. Vitamin $B_{12}$ content is 5μg per 100g. Vitamin C content is only 5mg per 100g.

---

**rose-hip syrup,** in undiluted form is a very rich source of vitamin C. Traces of vitamin E present. Traces only of thiamine, riboflavin, nicotinic acid, pyridoxine, pantothenic acid, folic acid and biotin. Vitamin C content is 295mg per 100ml.

---

**runner beans,** when boiled supply 400μg carotene per 100g and 0.5mg vitamin E. B vitamins present include (in mg per 100g): thiamine 0.03; riboflavin 0.07; nicotinic acid 0.8; pyridoxine 0.04; pantothenic acid 0.04. Useful source of folic acid at 28μg per 100g but only traces of biotin. Vitamin C present is 5mg per 100g when boiled, reduced from 20mg per 100g in the raw state, but better than canned runner beans at only 2mg per 100g.

---

**rutabagas,** virtually devoid of carotene and vitamin E. Supply B vitamins (in mg per 100g), in the raw and boiled states respectively, of: thiamine 0.06, 0.04; riboflavin 0.04, 0.03; nicotinic acid 1.4, 1.0; pyridoxine 0.20, 0.12; pantothenic acid 0.11, 0.07. Folic acid present is 27 and 21μg per 100g. Traces only of biotin. Good source of vitamin C, providing 25 and 17mg per 100g for raw and boiled vegetable respectively.

---

**rutin,** bioflavonoid, particularly rich in buckwheat. Used to treat bleeding gums and strengthen capillary walls at daily intakes of 60 to 600mg. Preferably taken with vitamin C (up to 500mg daily) at same time.

---

**rye flour,** less rich in B vitamins than whole wheat flour but still good source, providing (in mg per 100g): thiamine 0.40; riboflavin 0.22; nicotinic acid 2.6; pyridoxine 0.35; folic acid 0.078; pantothenic acid 1.0; biotin 0.006; vitamin E 1.5.

# S

**sago,** starch granules from the stem of Metroxylon *rumphii martius* or Metroxylon *sagu rottboell*, family palmae, commonly known as the sago-palm. Devoid of carotene and vitamin C but contains traces of vitamin E. Traces only of thiamine, riboflavin, nicotinic acid, pyridoxine, pantothenic acid, folic acid and biotin.

**salsify,** purple-flowered species of goat's-beard cultivated for its root, tasting like asparagus. Completely devoid of carotene and vitamin E. Some thiamine (0.03mg per 100g); nicotinic acid (0.3mg per 100g) that is derived from tryptophane; and vitamin C (4mg per 100g) is present.

**Savoy cabbage,** average level of carotene is 0.3mg per 100g but most of this is in the outer green leaves. Vitamin E also mainly in outer green leaves (7.0mg per 100g), but inner white leaves contain only 0.2mg. All B vitamins are reduced on boiling. Levels are as follows, raw figures first (in mg per 100g): thiamine 0.06, 0.03; riboflavin 0.05, 0.03; nicotinic acid 0.8, 0.4; pyridoxine 0.16, 0.10; pantothenic acid 0.21, 0.15. Folic acid (in µg per 100g) levels are 90, 35 for raw and boiled, but traces only of biotin. Drastic loss of vitamin C from 60 to 15mg per 100g when cabbage is boiled.

**scallions,** in the raw state provide traces only of carotene and vitamin E. Poor source of B vitamins apart from folic acid. Levels are (in mg per 100g): thiamine 0.03; riboflavin 0.05; nicotinic acid 0.4; pyridoxine 0.10; pantothenic acid 0.14. Useful folic acid content of 40µg per 100g but only 0.9µg biotin. Good source of vitamin C at average 25mg per 100g.

**Schilling test,** specific for detecting vitamin $B_{12}$ deficiency induced by non-absorption of vitamin from diet. Small amount of radioactive vitamin $B_{12}$ given by mouth followed some time later by high dose intravenously to flush out absorbed vitamin. Radioactivity in urine measured over 24 hours. Test repeated with radioactive vitamin plus intrinsic factor. Differences in two amounts excreted in urine allows diagnosis to be made.

---

**schizophrenia,** a group of mental disorders in people who exhibit: 1. disturbance of logical associations; 2. limited range of emotional response; 3. autism; 4. mixed feelings to an incapacitating degree. Has been treated with folic acid and pyridoxine or folic acid alone at high potencies. Others respond to nicotinamide plus vitamin C. Occasionally vitamin $B_{12}$ injections may help. *See* megavitamin therapy.

---

**scurvy,** disease specific to vitamin C deficiency. Symptoms are lassitude, weakness, irritability, vague muscle and joint pains, loss of weight, bleeding gums, gingivitis, loosening of the teeth. Minute hemorrhages under the skin followed by large hemorrhage in thigh muscles. Therapy with vitamin C at oral doses of 200-2000mg daily.

---

**seafood,** includes: crustacea such as crab, lobster, prawns, scampi and shrimps; and molluscs such as cockles, mussels, oysters, scallops, whelks and winkles. All contain traces only of vitamin A, carotene and vitamin D. Vitamin E levels vary from 0.1 to 1.5mg per 100g with lobster, mussels, oysters and whelks towards the upper end of the range.

Only moderate concentrations of the B vitamins are present in these seafoods and these are (in mg per 100g): thiamine 0.01-0.10; riboflavin 0.01-0.20; nicotinic acid 0.5-6.3; pyridoxine 0.03-0.35; pantothenic acid 0.06-1.63.

All seafoods provide vitamin $B_{12}$ at up to 2μg per 100g, but oysters are richest at a concentration of 15μg. Folic acid and biotin are present only in traces. Vitamin C is negligible in most of these seafoods, but the exceptions are Pacific oysters with 22mg per 100g and Olympia oysters with 38mg per 100g. *See also* Fish.

---

**seakale,** completely devoid of carotene and vitamin E. Some thiamine (0.06mg per 100g) and nicotinic acid (0.2mg per 100g) derived from tryptophane is present. Good source of vitamin C at 18mg per 100g.

---

**seasonal supplementation,**   extra vitamin A required during winter because of low environmental temperatures. Extra vitamin D required during winter because sunshine is shorter-lasting and weaker and body is more covered. Extra vitamin C required during winter because of prevalence of respiratory infections and intake of fresh fruit and vegetables in diet is decreased. Extra vitamin B complex should be taken during winter to help overcome stress of low environmental temperatures.

---

**seborrheic dermatitis,**   chronic, reddish, scaling inflammation of skin often occurring with acne, rosacea and psoriasis. In infants, responds to biotin therapy, 5mg daily until cured. In adults, sometimes responds to pyridoxine therapy with ointment of 10mg pyridoxine per gram base in addition to biotin given orally.

---

**selenium,**   trace mineral that has synergistic action with vitamin E. Usual ratio is 200IU vitamin with 25$\mu$g selenium. Has been used successfully as supplement in treatment of angina at dose rate of above ratio three times daily.

---

**Selye, Hans,**   medical professor at University of Montreal, Canada, who revolutionized medical thinking on stress and its effects on body nutrients and requirements of vitamins.

---

**semolina,**   starchy product derived from corn. Contains trace of vitamin E but no carotene or vitamin C. All figures are for the raw cereal and will be reduced on boiling because of water uptake. B vitamins present are (in mg per 100g): thiamine 0.10; riboflavin 0.02; nicotinic acid 2.9; pyridoxine 0.15; pantothenic acid 0.3. Useful folic acid levels of 25$\mu$g per 100g; biotin level of 1$\mu$g per 100g.

---

**senile dementia,**   due to a degenerative process with a large loss of cells from certain brain areas. Condition is more common in women and appears usually in seventh or eighth decade of life, i.e., later than Alzheimer's

Disease. For treatment *see* Alzheimer's Disease.

---

**sherry,** a fortified wine providing some B vitamins, the dry type bearing the highest concentrations. Traces only of carotene. B vitamins present are (in mg per 100g): thiamine, trace; riboflavin 0.1; nicotinic acid, range 0.07-0.10; pyridoxine 0.008-0.009; vitamin $B_{12}$ trace. Trace only of folic acid. All sherries are devoid of vitamin C.

---

**shingles,** acute infection of the central nervous system caused by a virus and characterized by skin blisters and pain in the nerve endings of the skin. Also known as herpes zoster.

Has been treated with vitamin C by injection at a dose of 3 grams every 12 hours plus one gram orally every two hours. Pain was relieved and blisters dried up within 72 hours. Some people respond to injections of vitamin $B_{12}$, 500µg daily, and are clear by third day. High oral doses of whole vitamin B complex recommended in all cases to help clear up nerve lesions. Continue after blisters have dried up. May also respond to high daily intakes (up to 3g daily) of amino acid L-lysine in addition to vitamin supplementation.

---

**Shute, Wilfred, E.,** cardiologist, Canadian, who founded Shute Institute for Laboratory and Clinical Medicine in London, Ontario, Canada, to study the treatment of heart disease with vitamin E.

---

**skin cancer,** *see* cancer.

---

**skin color,** dark pigmentation of skin reduces effect of ultra-violet light in producing vitamin D in the skin. Hence a long exposure to sunlight is necessary to produce sufficient vitamin D or ensure sufficient by eating D-rich foods or by supplementation.

---

**skin depigmentation,** *see* vitiligo.

---

**skin diseases,** sometimes related to mild deficiency of vitamins and some

162

will respond to oral intakes of vitamins plus direct application to skin. Vitamins particularly important to healthy skin are A, riboflavin, nicotinic acid, pyridoxine, biotin, C, E and F. *See* acne, dermatitis, eczema, seborrheic dermatitis, psoriasis.

---

**slimming,**   regimes that reduce daily calorie intake to 1000 calories or less will usually cause concomitant decrease in vitamin and mineral in diet to levels below recommended daily intake. Multivitamin and multimineral supplement essential on daily basis while slimming.

---

**smell,**   sense may be reduced by vitamin A deficiency; restored by intramuscular injection of high potencies of the vitamin.

---

**Smith, E. Lester,**   British scientist who was first to isolate vitamin $B_{12}$ from liver in 1948.

---

**smoking,**   *see* acetaldehyde and lung cancer.

---

**soups,**   all soups as eaten provide some B vitamins but little else apart from lentil and tomato soups which provide also vitamin A, carotene and vitamin D. All figures refer to canned, condensed as eaten and dried as eaten, soups. B vitamins present are (in mg per 100g) in the ranges quoted: thiamine 0.01-0.07; riboflavin 0.01-0.05; nicotinic acid 0.1-0.8; pyridoxone 0.01-0.07. Folic acid detected only in soups based on tomatoes and mushrooms and at levels of 2-12µg per 100g. Thiamine level of dried oxtail soup as eaten is 0.8mg per 100g which is mainly derived from the flavoring agent.

   *Lentil soup* provides also 40µg vitamin A per 100g; 430µg carotene per 100g and 0.28µg vitamin D per 100g, due mainly to ham ingredient plus traces of vitamin C.

   *Tomato soup* provides also 210µg carotene per 100g and traces of vitamin C.

---

**soy flour,**   excellent source of B vitamins that is even better when defatted providing (in mg per 100g): *Full fat* — thiamine 0.75; riboflavin 0.31;

nicotinic acid 10.6; pyridoxine 0.57; folic acid 0.40; pantothenic acid 1.8; biotin 0.7. *Defatted* — thiamine 0.90; riboflavin 0.36; nicotinic acid 13.0; pyridoxine 0.68; folic acid 0.43; pantothenic acid 2.1; biotin 0.07.

**spaghetti,**  pasta made from wheat flour. Provides no carotene or vitamin E. Trace of vitamin C in canned variety but this comes from the tomato sauce. Vitamins are reduced in concentration when the raw pasta is boiled or canned, mainly because of water uptake. B vitamins present (in mg per 100g), for raw, boiled and canned spaghetti respectively, are: thiamine 0.14, 0.01, 0.01; riboflavin 0.06, 0.01, 0.01; nicotinic acid 4.8, 1.2, 0.7; pyridoxine 0.06, 0.01, 0.01; pantothenic acid 0.3, trace, trace. Folic acid levels are respectively 13, 2 and 2μg per 100g; traces only of biotin.

**Spies, T.,**  American doctor who first demonstrated that folic acid from green leaves cured the anemia of pregnancy described by Dr. Lucy Wills fifteen years earlier.

**spinach,**  when boiled is an excellent source of carotene at 6.0mg per 100g (range 4-10mg); vitamin E content is 2.0mg per 100g. Levels of B vitamins are (in mg per 100g): thiamine 0.07; riboflavin 0.15; nicotinic acid 1.8; pyridoxine 0.18; pantothenic acid 0.21. Rich source of folic acid at 140μg per 100g but traces only of biotin (0.1μg per 100g).

**spirits,**  all alcoholic spirits are completely devoid of all vitamins.

**spironolactone,**  diuretic. Reduces availability of vitamin A.

**spirulina,**  blue-green alga, used as a staple food by the Aztecs of Mexico and now being developed as a high-protein food supplement rich in vitamins and minerals. The vitamins present are (in mg per 100g): carotene 250; vitamin E 19.0; thiamine 5.5; riboflavin 4.0; nicotinic acid 11.8; pyridoxine 0.3; pantothenic acid 1.1; inositol 35.0; folic acid 0.05; biotin 0.04; vitamin $B_{12}$ 0.2.

**split dried peas,**    losses occur in boiling and reduction in concentration due to uptake of water. Carotene level reduced from 150µg per 100g in dry state to 50µg when boiled, due to hydration. Levels of B vitamins for raw and boiled split peas respectively (in mg per 100g) are: thiamine 0.70, 0.11; riboflavin 0.20, 0.06; nicotinic acid 6.7, 2.3; pyridoxine 0.13, undetected; pantothenic acid 2.0, undetected. Folic acid levels are 33µg per 100g. Traces only of vitamin C.

**spring cabbage,**    when boiled supplies good amounts of carotene (0.5mg per 100g) but vitamin E level only 0.2mg. Levels of B vitamins (in mg per 100g) are: thiamine 0.03; riboflavin 0.03; nicotinic acid 0.4; pyridoxine 0.10; pantothenic acid 0.15. Some folic acid present at 50µg per 100g but negligible biotin. Supplies 25mg vitamin C per 100g.

**spring greens,**    when boiled supply good quantities of carotene at 4.0mg per 100g (range 1-10mg). Some vitamin E present (1.1mg per 100g). B vitamins present are (in mg per 100g): thiamine 0.06; riboflavin 0.20; nicotinic acid 0.8; pyridoxine 0.16; pantothenic acid 0.30. Good source of folic acid at 110µg per 100g; some biotin present (0.4µg per 100g). Excellent source of vitamin C with levels of 30mg per 100g (range 20-70mg).

**sprue,**    tropical disease characterized by sore mouth, fatty diarrhea and symptoms of malnutrition. Inability to absorb fat-soluble vitamins means supplementation of all must be by injection or orally as water-solubilized variety. Also needs for vitamin B complex.

**squash,**    poor source of B vitamins, reduced even further when boiled. Supplies 30µg carotene per 100g with only traces of vitamin E. Negligible levels of thiamine and riboflavin. Other B vitamins (in mg per 100g) supplied, by raw and boiled squash respectively, are: nicotinic acid 0.4, 0.3; pyridoxine 0.06, 0.03; pantothenic acid 0.10, 0.07. Folic acid content reduced from 13 to 6µg per 100g boiling.

**stamina,**    dependent on blood vitamin E levels. Russian claims that pangamic acid synergizes effect of vitamin E. *See* endurance.

**sterility,**  *see* fertility.

---

**steroids,**  *see* corticosteroids.

---

**stilboestrol,**  synthetic oestrogen. Reduces body levels of pyridoxine.

---

**stomatitis,**  inflammatory condition of the mouth which may occur as a primary disease or as a symptom of some other disease, e.g. sprue. May respond to daily intake of 300mg nicotinamide orally. *See also* glossitis, gingivitis.

---

**Stone, Irwin,**  American biochemist who introduced the concept of high vitamin C intakes for optimum health and influenced Linus Pauling in his development of orthomolecular medicine.

---

**strawberries,**  rich source of vitamin C and supply useful quantities of B vitamins. When fruit is canned there is some loss of vitamins especially vitamin C. Carotene contents for the raw and canned fruit are 30 and 2$\mu$g per 100g respectively. Vitamin E level in both is 0.2mg per 100g. B vitamins present are (in mg per 100g), for the raw and canned fruit respectively: thiamine 0.02, 0.01; riboflavin 0.03, 0.02; nicotinic acid 0.5, 0.4; pyridoxine 0.06, 0.03; pantothenic acid 0.34, 0.31. Folic acid levels (in $\mu$g per 100g) are 20 in both fresh and canned strawberries; biotin levels are stable at 1.1$\mu$g per 100g. Vitamin C content is 60mg (range 40-90mg) per 100g in fresh strawberries that is reduced to 21mg per 100g in the canned variety. Frozen strawberries have similar vitamin content to the fresh fruit but vitamin C content is reduced to 50mg per 100g.

---

**stress,**  increases body's requirements of vitamin B complex and particularly pantothenic acid because of its role in producing anti-stress hormones. Also vitamin C for the same reason. During stressful periods increase vitamin B complex and C intakes to ten-fold minimum daily requirements at least.

*Oxidative stress* — increase also vitamin E intake to at least 400IU daily. *See* vitamin E.

*Physical stress — see* athletes.

---

**stretch marks,**   also known as striae. Apply vitamin E cream as soon as possible and supplement diet with 400IU daily in divided doses.

---

**stroke,**   cerebrovascular disease due to atherosclerosis of brain blood-vessels and high blood-pressure.

Prevention or post-stroke treatment should include high intakes of vitamin E (400-600IU), vitamin C (500-1000mg), vitamin F (safflower oil or evening primrose oil, 3g daily), lecithin (5-15g daily), fish oils containing EPA and DHA (3g daily) and a switch from saturated dietary fats to polyunsaturated oils.

---

**suet,**   has animal fats as base and contains the following vitamins (in μg per 100g): vitamin A 52; carotene 73; nicotinic acid 200; vitamin E 1500. Traces of all the B vitamins but completely devoid of vitamin C.

---

**sugar,**   refined white variety is completely devoid of all vitamins.

*Demerara* sugar contains the following B vitamins in mg per 100g: thiamine, trace; riboflavin 0.01; nicotinic acid 2.0; pyridoxine 0.1; pantothenic acid 0.20mg. Contains also choline (2.8mg per 100g); inositol (24.0mg per 100g).

*Muscovado and light muscovado* sugars contain the following B vitamins in mg per 100g: thiamine 0.02; riboflavin 0.03; nicotinic acid 6.5; pyridoxine 0.06; pantothenic acid 0.8. Contains also choline (10.4mg per 100g); inositol (78mg per 100g).

---

**sulpha drugs,**   anti-infection drugs that function by inhibiting uptake of PABA by harmful bacteria. PABA should *not* be taken as supplement while taking sulpha drugs. Prevent synthesis of vitamin K by destroying intestinal bacteria.

---

**sulphasalazine,**   used to treat Crohn's disease and ulcerative colitis. Prevents absorption of folic acid.

---

**sulphitocobalamin,**   *see* $B_{12}$ vitamin.

---

**sulphonamides,**   *see* sulpha drugs.

---

**sultanas,**   golden seedless raisins, a dried form of certain types of grape so vitamin content is higher than original fruit with the exception of vitamin C, which is destroyed during the drying process. Carotene content is $30\mu g$ per 100g; vitamin E is present at a level of 0.7mg per 100g. B vitamins present are (in mg per 100g): thiamine 0.10; riboflavin 0.08; nicotinic acid 0.6; pyridoxine 0.30; pantothenic acid 0.10. Folic acid level is only $4\mu g$ per 100g; biotin has not been detected. Completely devoid of vitamin C.

---

**sunburn,**   vitamin E cream applied directly and take 600IU (200IU three times daily) orally to help healing and prevent scarring. Vitamin C (1000-1500mg daily) will help healing and prevent infection. In addition 15mg zinc daily will benefit.

---

**sunscreen agent,**   most effective is PABA which is incorporated at 5 per cent live in creams and lotions. Also may be best protectant against skin cancer induced by ultra-violet light.

---

**sunshine vitamin,**   *see* D vitamin.

---

**surgery,**   on intestinal tract may cause paralytic ileus (paralysis of the intestine) characterized by gas pains and abdominal distension. Doses of calcium pantothenate (50-100mg per day), preferably by injection, are used in prevention and treatment. Supplementary intakes of all vitamins but especially vitamin C (1000mg daily) and the mineral zinc (20mg daily) before and after surgery may help accelerate healing process. Post-surgical hemorrhage controlled by vitamin K given under medical supervision.

---

**sweet pickle,**   provides only thiamine, riboflavin and nicotinic acid at levels of 0.03, 0.01 and 0.3mg per 100g respectively.

---

**sweet potatoes,** excellent carotene content in yellow variety but traces only in the white. Both carotene and vitamin E are stable to boiling but some losses of the B vitamins. Carotene content is usually 4.0mg per 100g although some varieties contain 12.0mg per 100g. Contribute 4.0mg vitamin E per 100g. Levels of B vitamins in the raw and boiled vegetable respectively, are (in mg per 100g): thiamine 0.10, 0.08; riboflavin 0.06, 0.04; nicotinic acid 1.2, 0.9; pyridoxine 0.22, 0.13; pantothenic aid 0.94, 0.66. Folic acid levels are 52 and 25μg per 100g respectively. Biotin was not detected. Good source of vitamin C at 25 and 15mg per 100g respectively.

**sweetbread,** traces only of vitamins A, D, E and carotene. When fried supplies useful quantities of: riboflavin (0.24μg per 100g); nicotinic acid (6.2μ); vitamin $B_{12}$ (4μg per 100g). Small amounts only of other B vitamins and vitamin C.

**Szent-Gyorgy, Albert,** Hungarian doctor, winner of the Nobel Prize for his work in isolating vitamin C and the bioflavonoids.

# T

**tangerines,** the raw, edible portion is a good source of carotene and vitamin C with some B vitamins present, particularly folic acid. Carotene content is 100μg per 100g; vitamin E has not been detected. B vitamins present are (in mg per 100g): thiamine 0.07; riboflavin 0.02; nicotinic acid 0.3; pyridoxine 0.07; pantothenic acid 0.20. Good source of folic acid at 21μg per 100g; biotin has not been detected. Vitamin C content is 30mg per 100g edible portion.

**tapioca,** starch derivative of the tubers of cassava, also known as manioc. In the raw state there is no carotene or vitamin C in tapioca. Trace only of vitamin E. Traces only of thiamine, riboflavin, nicotinic acid, pyridoxine, pantothenic acid, folic acid and biotin.

---

**tea,**  dried leaf (Indian) has useful content of some vitamins but these are drastically reduced when it is infused. Traces only of carotene and vitamin C in dried leaf but not detectable in the drink. B vitamins present are (in mg per 100g), for the dried leaf and infusion respectively: thiamine 0.14, trace; riboflavin 1.2, 0.01; nicotinic acid 7.5, 0.1; pantothenic acid 1.3, trace.

---

**teeth,**  pyridoxine may help prevent tooth decay, particularly in children, when taken at a daily dose of 10mg. Vitamins A and D essential during childhood for normal development of healthy teeth. Vitamin C, at intakes of 100mg with each meal, has been used as orthodontic supplement in children. *See also* bruxism.

---

**temperature,**  *see* seasonal supplementation.

---

**tetracycline,**  antibiotic. Prevents formation of vitamin K by intestinal bacteria.

---

**thiamin(e),**  *see* B$_1$ vitamin.

---

**thrombophlebitis,**  *see* phlebitis.

---

**thrombosis,**  *see* blood clot.

---

**thymus,**  gland concerned with development of immune system and resistance to infection. Fully developed at 2 years of age then slowly regressive after a period of stagnation. Full activity requires adequate vitamin A, choline, folic acid, vitamin B$_{12}$ and amino acid. Methionine essential in pregnant mother for full, efficient development of thymus in baby.

---

**tobacco amblyopia,**   *see* eyes.

---

**tocopherol,**   E vitamin.

---

**tomato juice,**   canned variety is a rich source of carotene with useful amounts of B vitamins and vitamin C. Carotene content is 500µg per 100g; 0.2mg vitamin E per 100g also present. B vitamins present are (in mg per 100g): thiamine 0.06; riboflavin 0.03; nicotinic acid 0.8; pyridoxine 0.11; pantothenic acid 0.20. Folic acid is 13µg per 100g; that of biotin is 1µg per 100g. Vitamin C content is 20mg per 100g.

---

**tomato purée,**   very rich source of carotene and vitamin C, proiding also some useful quantities of B vitamins. Carotene content is 2.86mg per 100g; vitamin E present is 6.9mg per 100g. B vitamins present are (in mg per 100g): thiamine 0.34; riboflavin 0.17; nicotinic acid 4.8; pyridoxine 0.63; pantothenic acid 1.1. Good source of folic acid at 140µg per 100g; and of biotin at 8µg per 100g. Vitamin C content is 100mg per 100g.

---

**tomato sauce,**   good source of carotene and some B vitamins and vitamin C. Carotene content is 1.23mg per 100g; vitamin E level is 1.4mg per 100g. No vitamins A and D present if recipe does not include animal products. B vitamins present are (in mg per 100g): thiamine 0.08; riboflavin 0.05; nicotinic acid 1.4; pyridoxine 0.11; pantothenic acid 0.3. Folic acid level is 15µg per 100g; biotin level is 2µg per 100g. Vitamin C content is 10mg per 100g.

---

**tomatoes,**   raw tomatoes contain highest quantity of vitamins but little lost in canning. Carotene contents (in µg per 100g) of raw and canned varieties are respectively 600 (range 200-1000) and 500 (range 300-600). Vitamin E level constant at 1.4mg per 100g. Levels of B vitamins are (in mg per 100g), for raw and canned tomatoes respectively: thiamine 0.06, 0.06; riboflavin 0.04, 0.03; nicotinic acid 0.8, 0.8; pyridoxine 0.11, 0.11; pantothenic acid 0.2, 0.2. Folic acid levels are (in µg per 100g) 25 and 20 respectively; those of biotin are 1.5 and 1.5. Vitamin C contents are 20 (range 10-30) and 18mg per 100g respectively.

*Fried* tomatoes contain only 10mg vitamin C per 100g.

---

**tongue,**   supplies only traces of vitamins A, D and carotene. Vitamin E levels vary from 0.21 to 0.35mg per 100g. Good source of the B vitamins, providing (in mg per 100g): thiamine 0.06-0.17; riboflavin 0.29-0.49; nicotinic acid 7.6-9.8; pyridoxine 0.10-0.18; pantothenic acid 0.5-1.0. Good levels of vitamin $B_{12}$, at 4-7µg per 100g, but traces only of folic acid and biotin. Small amounts (2-7mg per 100g) of vitamin C present.

---

**torula yeast,**   torulopsis utilis. Strain of yeast less bitter than baker's and brewer's varieties containing the following vitamins (in mg per 100g dried product): carotene (trace); thiamine (15.0); riboflavin (5.0); pyridoxine (3.5); nicotinic acid (50.0); pantothenic acid (10.0); biotin (0.1); folic acid (3.0). Rich source of RNA and DNA; together account for 12 per cent of dried yeast.

---

**toxemia of pregnancy,**   may be related in some cases to lack of pyridoxine and more importantly folic acid.

---

**travel sickness,**   *see* nausea.

---

**toxic reactions,**   undesirable effects of vitamin therapy are rare in the West but they have been observed, usually as a result of excessive intake of vitamins when self-administered as supplements.

For the water-soluble vitamins it is difficult to produce high tissue levels because the kidneys readily excrete the excess when blood concentrations are above a certain threshold. There is no evidence that the body is able to convert excessive quantities of the B complex into their metabolically active forms above those normally present.

Fat-soluble vitamins, however, tend to be stored both in the liver and in the fatty tissues of the body. When these vitamins spill over into the tissues, toxic reactions occur and certain symptoms become apparent, summarized as follows:

*Vitamin A* — first indications of acute vitamin A toxicity were reported when seamen and Arctic explorers ate polar-bear liver which is a particularly rich source of the vitamin. Symptoms included drowsiness, increased cerebrospinal fluid (which bathes the spinal column and brain) pressure, vomiting and extensive peeling of the skin. Vitamin A quantities measured in millions of units were eaten.

At least twenty cases of children under three years of age with vitamin A poisoning have been described in USA medical literature. The cause was usually misguided enthusiasm on the part of the mothers who gave their offspring from 30mg (90 000IU) to 150mg (450 000IU) of vitamin A daily for several months. The symptoms of these chronic intakes included loss of appetite, irritability, a dry, itching skin, coarse, sparse hair and swellings over the long bones. Usually an enlarged liver was present.

Much of our knowledge of vitamin A toxicity comes from India and the Philippines where doses of 200 000IU are given to deficient patients in outlying villages once every six months. From 3-4 per cent of them suffer loss of appetite, nausea, vomiting and headache within 24 hours. These side-effects last only a few days, then as the body distributes the vitamin, deficiency symptoms disappear and the beneficial effects of the vitamins are felt.

Severe overdosage gives rise to generalized itching, redness of the skin, dry scaling of the skin and mucous membranes, cracking of the corners of the mouth and lips, inflamed tongue and gums, ulceration of the mouth and loss of hair. In addition there are fatigue, hemorrhages, retention of water, tenderness of the long bones and a tender enlarged liver. If intake is continued there is mental irritability, sleep disturbance, loss in weight and rises in the blood enzyme alkaline phosphatase which leads to calcium deposition in the blood-vessels.

Toxicity is unlikely if the daily intake is kept below 5000IU per kg body weight (i.e., 350 000IU for a 70kg or 11 stone individual) for not more than 200 days. Intervals of 4 to 6 weeks between courses of treatment are recommended. These levels of intakes apply only when the vitamin is being used therapeutically and under medical supervision. There is now an increased tendency to give large daily doses of vitamin A and its analogues for skin diseases and for cancer. The symptoms mentioned above apply mainly to vitamin A alcohol (retinol) because it is stored in the liver. Retinoic acid is not stored and is used where high blood levels are needed quickly.

Synthetic retinoic acid analogues (retinoids) can induce toxicity symptoms but at intakes higher than those of vitamin A. The widely used 13-cis-retinoic acid used to treat acne gives side-effects confined to the skin, the mucous membranes of the mouth, the nose and the eyes. Toxic symptoms rapidly abate when treatment with the analogues is stopped. Reducing the intake of vitamin A and its analogues is the only treatment for overdosage.

*Vitamin D* — there is a narrow gap between the nutrient requirement and the toxic dose. As little as five times the recommended intake (50µg daily) taken over prolonged periods can lead to high blood calcium levels in infants and calcium deposition in the kidneys of adults.

Toxicity is more likely in children, either because of excessive doses administered by over-zealous mothers or because of increased sensitivity of some infants to fortified milk containing the vitamin. The usual signs in children are loss of appetite with nausea and vomiting. Excessive passing of urine with consequent thirst are soon evident. Constipation often alternates with diarrhea. Frequently there are pains in the head and in the bones. The child becomes thin, irritable and depressed, eventually becoming stupored. Calcium deposits are laid down in the arteries, kidneys, heart, lungs and other soft tissues and organs. Death can result.

In adults a regular intake of more than 100 000IU (2.5mg) of vitamin D for long periods is required to produce the typical symptoms of weakness, nausea, vomiting, constipation, excessive passing of urine, thirst, and dehydration. Less obvious but more serious results are deposition of calcium in the soft tissues and organs and eventually kidney failure leading to death.

High doses of vitamin D are used in treating metabolic bone disease, hypoparathyroidism, malabsorption and certain arthritic conditions. Potent preparations must be taken for long periods so close medical monitoring is essential.

The only treatment for vitamin D overdosage is to stop taking the vitamin.

*Vitamin E* — the only side-effect noted with this vitamin is muscle weakness in a few people taking at least 600IU daily. Many more have taken from 400 to 1600IU daily with no ill-effects. In a period spanning forty years, doctors at the Shute Institite in Canada have treated over 40000 patients with doses of vitamin E up to 5000IU daily with no discernible side-effects. Occasionally there is a transient rise in blood-pressure in susceptible people given over 800IU daily but no effect has been noted in those being treated for high blood-pressure. Both muscle weakness and the raised blood-pressure quickly disappear when the vitamin intake is stopped or reduced to 400IU daily. Occasionally contact dermatitis has occurred when people applied the pure oil to the skin or even an ointment or cream containing more than 100IU per gram. Reduction of the potency removes the allergic reaction.

*Thiamine* — very occasionally injections of thiamine can cause hypersensitivity reactions in susceptible people. Effects include itching and swelling at the site of injection; swelling of the tongue, lips and eyes; generalized itching and sweating; sneezing, wheezing, difficulty in breathing and cyanosis (where the skin becomes blue); nausea; low blood-pressure and, very rarely, death has resulted. No side-effects have been reported from orally-administered thiamine.

*Nicotinic acid* — large doses of between 3 and 10 grams daily have been prescribed to reduce blood cholesterol levels and the toxic reactions include flushing of the skin of the face, neck and chest accompanied by itching in these areas. More than one-third of patients so treated continue to suffer this flushing while undergoing this therapy. In some there are rashes, dry skin and increased pigmentation of the skin. Occasionally jaundice appears, accompanied by nausea, diarrhea, abdominal pain and headache in as many as 20 to 40 per cent of patients treated. Gastric and duodenal ulcers can worsen.

Nicotinamide in similar doses does not cause flushing but liver damage has been recorded. Nicotinic acid must therefore be used with caution and under close monitoring in those suffering from gastric and duodenal ulcers, gout, diabetes and liver disease and in pregnant women.

*Pyridoxine* — until recently was believed to be non-toxic, although for some time it has been known to neutralize the effect of the drug levodopa used in treating Parkinson's disease.

Daily intakes of at least 2000mg pyridoxine taken over 2 to 40 months have given rise to peripheral neuropathy in seven subjects. Typical symptoms started with numbness in the feet and unstable gait. This led to increasing inability to walk steadily, particularly in the dark, and difficulty in handling small objects. Numbness and clumsiness of the hands followed within months, sufficient to impair typing ability; there were also changes in the feeling in lips and tongue. Normal blood plasma levels of pyridoxine are in the range of 0.36 to 1.8µg per 100ml but those patients had levels of 3.0µg and above. After one month's abstinence from pyridoxine supplementation, the level fell to 1.7µg per 100ml plasma. In all cases, withdrawal of pyridoxine led to improvement in symptoms and tests indicated a marked recovery of the nervous system, but the process took several months. None of these patients experienced symptoms when their intake was below 2000mg pyridoxine daily. There is no evidence of harm from the more usual daily dose of 25 to 100mg taken for PMT.

*Folic acid* — antagonism has been reported between folic acid and the drug phenytoin used in treating epilepsy. Hence balance between drug and vitamin is critical and best left to the medical practitioner.

High folic acid intakes can deplete vitamin $B_{12}$ stores in the body. If given to those suffering from pernicious anemia resulting from malabsorption of vitamin $B_{12}$, high-dose folic acid can mask the blood anemia symptoms but allow the spinal column nerve degeneration to continue. Hence the importance of diagnosing megaloblastic anemia as due to either folic acid or vitamin $B_{12}$ deficiency.

Oral therapy has given rise to loss of appetite, abdominal distension and flatulence. Occasionally injection of folic acid can cause transient rise in temperature and symptoms of fever.

*Vitamin $B_{12}$* — toxicity reactions from oral dosage have never been reported. Very rare allergic reactions have occurred following intramuscular injection of the vitamin.

*Riboflavin* — no reported toxicity reactions.

*Pantothenic acid* — no reported toxicity reactions even after long-term treatment with up to 2 grams daily in cases of rheumatoid arthritis, either orally or by injection.

*Carotene* — generally accepted as safe, even at intakes sufficient to impart a yellow color to the skin.

*Biotin* — no adverse reactions reported even in infants given 5mg daily, orally or by injection, for skin lesions.

*Vitamin C* — generally regarded as one of the safest vitamins, even when taken in massive doses. There are some who should avoid large (i.e., greater than 1g daily) intakes of the vitamin because they suffer from inherited metabolic diseases giving rise to excess oxalic acid, cystine or uric acid in the blood and urine. They have a greater tendency to form kidney stones. Such disease is rare and most people can tolerate vitamin C intakes up to 3g daily and even more. Those who suffer from kidney stones and those who are taking oral anticoagulant drugs should take high-dose vitamin C with caution although intakes of up to 500mg daily can be tolerated by these people for long periods.

Physical signs of overdose are gastro-intestinal and include nausea, abdominal cramps and diarrhea. The vitamin can also act as a diuretic causing increased urination but this can be beneficial in removing excess body water. If a high intake causes diarrhea, reducing the amount taken by 500mg or 1g daily will often reduce the side-effect. Previous claims that high vitamin C intakes can destroy vitamin $B_{12}$ have now been discounted.

**tretinoin,**　vitamin A acid; retinoic acid. Toxic effects include transitory stinging, redness, allergic dermatitis when applied to skin.

**triamterene,**　diuretic. Impairs folic acid utilization.

**trifluoperazine,**　antidepressant, bronchospasm relaxant, gastrointestinal sedative, sedative, anti-nausea agent. Prevents absorption of vitamin $B_{12}$.

**trigeminal neuralgia,**　severe, brief, lancing pain at either side of face. Known also as facial neuralgia. Has been relieved with large doses of thiamine (50-600mg daily).

**tripe,**　supplies very small quantities of all B vitamins with negligible amounts of vitamins A, D, carotene, E and C.

**tryptophan(e),**　essential amino acid normally supplied by the diet. Has been used to treat depression in high doses along with nicotinamide, pyridoxine and vitamin C. Precursor of nicotinic acid; 60mg tryptophane necessary for each mg of vitamin. Tryptophane in diet will not be sufficient to supply all nicotinic acid needs but conversion depends upon adequate quantities of thiamine, riboflavin, pyridoxine and biotin. Precursor of serotonin, an essential factor for nerve and brain function. Vitamin $B_6$ required for synthesis of serotinin, lack of which produces depression. Has been used to treat insomnia.

**turkey,**　when cooked supplies only traces of vitamins A, D, E and carotene. Concentrations of B vitamins (in mg per 100g) are: thiamine 0.07-0.10; riboflavin 0.11-0.29; nicotinic acid 3.8-15.6; pyridoxine 0.30-0.59; pantothenic acid 0.7-0.9; (in μg per 100g) vitamin $B_{12}$ 1-3; folic acid 8-25; biotin 1-2.
　Completely devoid of vitamin C. *See also* Meats: Cooking losses.

**turnip greens,**　when boiled excellent source of carotene at 6.0mg (range

4.0-12.0mg) per 100g. Vitamin E present at 1.0mg per 100g. B vitamins present (in mg per 100g) are: thiamine 0.06; riboflavin 0.20; nicotinic acid 0.9; pyridoxine 0.16; pantothenic acid 0.30. Good source of folic acid at 110μg per 100g; but only 0.4μg biotin present. Very good source of vitamin C at 40mg per 100g (range 20-70mg).

---

**turnips,**  completely devoid of carotene and vitamin E. B vitamins present (in mg per 100g), in the raw and boiled vegetable respectively, are: thiamine 0.04, 0.03; riboflavin 0.05, 0.04; nicotinic acid 0.8, 0.6; pyridoxine 0.11, 0.06; pantothenic acid 0.20, 0.14. Folic acid levels are 20 and 10μg per 100g respectively. Traces only of biotin. Good source of vitamin C with contents of 25 and 17mg per 100g respectively for raw and boiled variety.

---

# U

---

**ubiquinone,**  vitamin-like substance found in all body cells but particularly rich in heart muscle. Functions as oxygen transfer coenzyme. Synthesis dependent on vitamin E. Rich source is yeast. Known also as coenzyme Q.

---

**ulcers,**  open sores on the surface of the skin or mucous membranes.

*Decubitus — See* bedsores.

*Indolent* — one that will not heal. May respond to oral vitamin E (400-600IU daily) plus direct application of vitamin E cream.

*Leg* — sometimes associated with diabetes. Treat as for indolent with vitamin E *or* folic acid, 5mg tablets three times daily and in serious cases with additional injections of 20mg twice weekly.

*Gastric* — has responded to 150 000IU vitamin A daily for four weeks. *See also* digestive tract and vitamin U.

*Mouth* — prevented by adequate intakes of riboflavin (10mg daily) plus vitamin A (7500IU daily). May be treated by same regime. *See also* herpes simplex.

*Varicose — see indolent ulcer.*

---

# V

---

**varicose veins,** swollen, knotted and dilated condition of vein. *Bioflavonoids* (1000mg daily) plus vitamin C (500mg daily) can help reduce condition. *Vitamin E* (400-600IU) daily can reduce swelling, pain and prevent phlebitis. *Lecithin* (5-15g) daily complements action of vitamin E.

---

**veal,** when cooked all cuts supply only traces of vitamins A, D, E and carotene. Poor source of biotin and folic acid. Other B vitamins present (in mg per 100g) are in the range: thiamine 0.06-0.10; riboflavin 0.25-0.27; nicotinic acid 6.7-13.7; pyridoxine 0.30-0.32; pantothenic acid 0.5-0.6; (in $\mu$g per 100g) vitamin $B_{12}$ 1.0; folic acid 4-5.

Higher potencies associated with leaner cuts. Completely devoid of vitamin C. *See also* Meats: Cooking losses.

---

**veganism,** extreme form of vegetarianism where no product of animal, fish, fowl or insect is eaten. Practitioners, or vegans, may be prone to vitamin $B_{12}$ deficiency but this can be obtained from supplements which contain the vitamin produced by fermentation. Spirulina, an alga, can supply sufficient $B_{12}$ acceptable to vegans. Possible vitamin D deficiency overcome by exposure of skin to sunshine or supplements containing the vitamin derived from yeast.

---

**vegetables,** completely devoid of vitamin A, but some are good source of its precursor carotene. They contain no vitamin D but usually some vitamin E. Most supply all the B vitamins except for vitamin $B_{12}$, but concentrations vary. Some vegetables supply good quantities of vitamin C. Carotene and vitamin E are unaffected by cooking methods. Invariably some loss of B vitamins when vegetables are cooked. *See* individual varieties.

---

**vegetarianism,** practised by those who eat no meat, fish or fowl. May benefit from vitamin $B_{12}$ supplementation but probably obtain enough from dairy products in diet. Same source for vitamin D. Tend to receive high intakes of folic acid and vitamin C because of dietary habits.

---

**vermouth,** a fortified wine containing herbal extracts. Nicotinic acid content is 0.04mg per 100ml. Pyridoxine content is 0.004 (sweet) and 0.008 (dry) mg per 100ml. Traces only of thiamine, riboflavin, folic acid and vitamin $B_{12}$. All vermouths are completely devoid of vitamin C.

---

**veruccae,** *see* warts.

---

**virus,** the smallest of parasites. Consists of central core of nucleic acid and an outer cover of protein. Wholly dependent on bacterial, plant or animal cells for reproduction. Nucleic acid represents basic infective material. Best natural defences against viruses are adequate vitamin A and vitamin C. Viral infections best supplemented with vitamin A (7500IU) and vitamin C (up to 6g daily).

---

**vitamin,** derived from "vita" (meaning life) and "amine" (substance incorrectly assigned to all vitamins). Term first used by Polish chemist Casimir Funk in 1911. Micronutrient essential for health that cannot be synthesized in sufficient amounts by the animal or human body. Divided into fat soluble — A, D, E, F and K — and water-soluble — B-complex, C and P.

Vitamins must satisfy three criteria:

1. adequate amounts supplied only in the diet;
2. deficiency produces discrete clinical symptoms and disease;
3. disease and symptoms cured only with specific vitamin.

Exceptions may be vitamin D (produced in skin by sunshine) and biotin and vitamin K produced by intestinal bacterial synthesis.

---

**vitamin $B_3$,** nicotinic acid.

---

**vitamin B$_4$,**   adenine (no longer regarded as a vitamin).

**vitamin B$_5$,**   pantothenic acid.

**vitamin B$_7$,**   growth factor for micro-organisms but not for man.

**vitamin B$_8$,**   growth factor for micro-organisms but not for man.

**vitamin B$_9$,**   growth factor for micro-organisms but not for man.

**vitamin B$_{10}$,**   unidentified growth and feathering factor for chicks.

**vitamin B$_{11}$,**   unidentified growth and feathering factor for chicks.

**vitamin B$_{13}$,**   orotic acid.

**vitamin B$_{14}$,**   derivative of vitamin B$_{12}$.

**vitamin Bc,**   folic acid.

**vitamin BT,**   carnitine (no longer regarded as a vitamin).

**vitamin Bx,**   para-aminobenzoic acid.

**vitamin F,**   polyunsaturated fatty acids.

**vitamin G,**   B$_2$ vitamin.

**vitamin H,** biotin.

---

**vitamin H$_3$,** procaine (no longer regarded as a vitamin).

---

**vitamin L$_1$,** ortho-aminobenzoic acid; **L$_2$,** adenine derivative. Factors presumably necessary for lactation. Very doubtful significance in human beings.

---

**vitamin M,** folic acid.

---

**vitamin P,** bioflavonoids.

---

**vitamin PP,** nicotinic acid.

---

**vitamin T,** also known as tegotin, termitin, factor T, vitamin T Goetsch, Goetsch's vitamin. Complex of growth-promoting substances, originally obtained from termites. Also present in yeasts and fungi. Probably a mixture of known vitamins and growth-promoting factors but never characterized fully.

---

**vitamin U,** the anti-ulcer vitamin reported in cabbage leaves and other green vegetables. Believed to be L-methionine methylsulphonium salt. Has been used to treat gastric ulcers.

---

**vitiligo,** depigmentation of areas of skin which have lost ability to produce natural pigment melanin. Condition worsens on exposure to sunlight probably because non-affected areas become darker with tanning. Harmless condition apart from cosmetic blemish.

Has been treated with PABA, 50mg by injection twice daily plus 100mg twice a day orally. Condition improved after 6 to 8 months. May be complemented with additional pantothenic acid, vitamin B$_6$, zinc and manganese to stimulate melanin production.

---

# W

**Wald, George,** American scientist at Harvard University who first demonstrated relationship of vitamin A to vision.

---

**walnuts,** kernels are a good source of B vitamins with good quantities of vitamin E present. Vitamin E content is 18.8mg per 100g. B vitamins present are (in mg per 100g): thiamine 0.30; riboflavin 0.13; nicotinic acid 3.0; pyridoxine 0.73; pantothenic acid 0.9. Good folic acid level at 66μg per 100g; biotin level is 2.0μg per 100g. Ripe walnut kernels contain traces only of vitamin C but unripe kernels are very rich source at levels of 1200-1300mg per 100g.

---

**warfarin,** anti-coagulant drug. Acts by inhibiting action of vitamin K.

---

**warts,** common, benign skin eruptions caused by a virus. *See also* veruccae. Have been treated with directly applied solutions of water-solubilized vitamin A palmitate. Alternatively may respond to vitamin E oil applied directly plus oral supplement of 400IU daily.

---

**watercress,** when raw is good source of carotene at 3.0mg per 100g (range 1.5-3.5mg). Some vitamin E present (1.0mg per 100g). B vitamins present are (in mg per 100g): thiamine 0.10; riboflavin 0.10; nicotinic acid 1.1; pyridoxine 0.13; pantothenic acid 0.10. Excellent source of folic acid at 200μg per 100g with 0.4μg of biotin present. Very good source of vitamin C at 60mg per 100g (range 40-80mg).

---

**wheat germ,** germ or embryo of the wheat grain situated at the lower end; consists of root and shoot. Makes up 3 per cent of total weight of grain. Claimed that wheat germ (60g, or 2 ounces, daily) plus vitamin C (2000mg daily) more effective in preventing respiratory complaints than vitamin C alone. Usually stabilized by mild heat but final product still an excellent source of B and E vitamins, providing (in mg per 100g): thiamine 1.45; riboflavin 0.61; nicotinic acid 11.1; pyridoxine 0.95; folic acid 0.33; pantothenic acid 1.7; vitamin E 11.0.

**wheat-germ oil,**   expressed or solvent-extracted oil from germ of wheat grain. Rich source of vitamin E (190mg per 100g) and vitamin F (41.54g per 100g).

**whey factor,**   *see* orotic acid.

**white cabbage,**   in the raw state is practically devoid of carotene with little vitamin E (0.2mg per 100g). Levels of B vitamins (in mg per 100g) are: thiamine 0.06; riboflavin 0.05; nicotinic acid 0.6; pyridoxine 0.16; pantothenic acid 0.21. Some folic acid at 26$\mu$g per 100g but negligible biotin. Provides 40mg vitamin C per 100g.

**white currants,**   vitamin content comparable to that of red currants except that only traces of carotene are present. Vitamin E level is only 0.1mg per 100g. B vitamins present are (in mg per 100g), for raw and stewed white currants respectively: thiamine 0.04, 0.03; riboflavin 0.06, 0.05; nicotinic acid 0.3, 0.3; pyridoxine 0.05, 0.03; pantothenic acid 0.06, 0.05. Biotin levels are 2.6 and 2.0$\mu$g per 100g for raw and stewed fruit respectively. Folic acid too small to be detected. Good source of vitamin C at levels of 40 and 30mg per 100g for raw and stewed fruit respectively.

**white flour,**   unfortified contains many fewer B vitamins and vitamin E than whole-wheat, providing (in mg per 100g): thiamine 0.01; riboflavin 0.03; nicotinic acid 3.0; pyridoxine 0.15; folic acid 0.031; pantothenic acid 0.3; biotin 0.001; vitamin E trace. At present, white flour is fortified with thiamine and nicotinic acid to give values of 0.31 and 4.3 respectively but fortification may not be compulsory after 1985.

**white sugar,**   completely devoid of all vitamins.

**whole-grain flour,** usually whole-wheat, rich source of B vitamins providing (in mg per 100g): thiamine 0.46; riboflavin 0.08; nicotinic acid 8.1; pyridoxine 0.50; folic acid 0.057; pantothenic acid 0.8; biotin 0.007; vitamin E 2.1. Devoid of vitamins A, D, C and carotene.

---

**Williams, Roger J.,** American scientist, pioneer in the field of vitamin research and noted for discovering pantothenic acid.

---

**Wills, Lucy,** *see* Spies, T.

---

**wines,** red wines provide more B vitamins than rosé or white. Traces only of carotene in all types of wine. B vitamins present are (in mg per 100ml): thiamine, traces only; riboflavin 0.01-0.02; nicotinic acid 0.06-0.09; pantothenic acid 0.03-0.04; pyridoxine 0.012-0.023; vitamin $B_{12}$ traces. Traces only of folic acid; biotin appears to be absent. All wines are devoid of vitamin C.

---

**winter cabbage,** good source of carotene at 0.3mg per 100g. Outer green leaves contain 7.0mg per 100g but only 0.2mg in inner leaves. Carotene and vitamin E levels unaffected by boiling. All B vitamins are reduced by boiling. Levels are as follows, raw figures first (in mg per 100g): thiamine 0.06, 0.03; riboflavin 0.05, 0.03; nicotinic acid 0.8, 0.5; pyridoxine 0.16, 0.10; pantothenic acid 0.21, 0.15. Folic acid reduced on boiling from 90μg to 35μg per 100g. Negligible biotin levels. Vitamin C concentration reduced from 55 to 20mg per 100g on boiling.

---

**women,** have different vitamin and mineral needs to men because of menstrual cycle. May have requirements for pyridoxine ten days or so before menstruation far above those supplied by the diet. Usually minimum of 25mg daily. Extra needs for vitamin C, folic acid, vitamin $B_{12}$ and vitamin E to ensure maximum incorporation of iron into hemoglobin to replace blood losses of menstrual flow. Extra requirements of all vitamins and minerals while pregnant and during period of breast feeding. Those taking contraceptive pill have increased requirements for certain vitamins. *See also* contraceptives and menstruation.

---

**wound healing,** accelerated by supplementary intakes of vitamin C, vitamin E, vitamin A and mineral zinc.

# X

**xerophthalmia,** drying and degenerative disease of the transparent part of the eye associated with vitamin A deficiency.

# Y

**yam,** some carotene present in the raw and boiled states (both 12µg per 100g) but vitamin E virtually absent. B vitamins present (in mg per 100g) are, for the raw and boiled variety respectively: thiamine 0.10, 0.05; riboflavin 0.03, 0.01; nicotinic acid 0.8, 0.8; pyridoxine, absent; pantothenic acid 0.63, 0.44. Traces only of folic aid (6µg per 100g) but biotin was not detected. Some vitamin C present but most lost on boiling (from 10mg to 2mg per 100g).

**yeast extract,** concentrate made from vegetables, usually including brewer's yeast. Very rich source of most of the B vitamins but completely devoid of carotene, vitamin E and vitamin C. B vitamins present are (in mg per 100g): thiamine 3.1; riboflavin 11; nicotinic acid 67; pyridoxine 1.3. Folic acid level is 1010µg per 100g; vitamin $B_{12}$ content is 0.5µg per 100g but this is probably added. *See also* brewer's yeast.

**yogurt,** useful source of some B vitamins plus fat-soluble variety. Higher potencies than milk because of bacterial synthesis, providing (in mg per

100g): vitamin A 0.008; carotene 0.005; thiamine 0.05; riboflavin 0.26; nicotinic acid 1.16; pyridoxine 0.04; folic acid 0.002; vitamin E 0.03; vitamin $B_{12}$ trace; vitamin D trace.

# Bibliography

*A Guide to the Vitamins.* John Marks, MTP Press, Lancaster, 1979

*Cancer and Vitamin C.* E. Cameron and L. Pauling, The Linus Pauling Institute of Science and Medicine, USA, 1979

*Human Nutrition and Dietetics.* S. Davidson, R. Passmore, J. F. Brock and A. S. Trusswell, Churchill Livingstone, Edinburgh, 7th edition 1979;

*The Complete Book of Vitamins.* Rodale Press, Emmaus, USA, 1979

*The Complete, Updated Vitamin E Book.* Wilfred E. Shute, Keats Publishing, New Canaan, Connecticut, 1975

*The Composition of Foods.* A. A. Paul and A. T. Southgate, HMSO, London, 4th edition 1978

*The Importance of Vitamins to Human Health.* ed. T. G. Taylor, MTP Press, Lancaster, 1979

*Vitamin C (Ascorbic Acid).* J. N. Counsell and D. M. Hornig, Applied Science Publishers, London, 1981

*Vitamin C, the Common Cold and the Flu.* Linus Pauling, W. H. Freeman and Company, San Francisco, 1976

The following periodicals:

*Adverse Drug Reaction Bulletin*
*American Journal of Clinical Nutrition*
*British Journal of Nutrition*
*British Journal of Pharmacology*
*British Medical Journal*
*International Journal for Vitamin and Nutrition Research*
*International Journal of Vitaminology*
*Journal of Alternative Medicine*
*Journal of Atherosclerosis Research*
*Journal of Clinical Pathology*
*Journal of Nutrition*

# THE DICTIONARY OF VITAMINS

*Journal of Paediatrics*
*Journal of the American Medical Association*
*New England Journal of Medicine*
*Nutrition Metabolism*
*The Lancet*
*The Practitioner*
*Vitamins and Hormones*